NEBRASKA ISOLATION & QUARANTINE MANUAL

Edited by

Theodore J. Cieslak
Mark G. Kortepeter
Christopher J. Kratochvil
James V. Lawler

Library of Congress Cataloging-in-Publication Data
Names: University of Nebraska Press, issuing body.
Title: Nebraska isolation & quarantine manual.
Other titles: Nebraska isolation and quarantine manual
Description: Lincoln, Nebraska: University of Nebraska Press, [2019] |
Includes bibliographical references.
Identifiers: LCCN 2019018737 | ISBN 9780989353731 (pbk.: alk. paper)
Subjects: | MESH: Quarantine—methods | Patient Isolation—methods |
Communicable Disease Control
Classification: LCC SB985.N43 | NLM WA 230 | DDC 614.4/6—dc23 LC
record available at https://lccn.loc.gov/2019018737

Cover design by Lacey Losh.

The yellow-and-black checked flag depicted on the cover is an international maritime signal flag denoting the letter "L" or "Lima." When flown from a ship, it has been used to indicate that the vessel is under quarantine. The "Q" or "Quebec" flag is solid yellow; while it was apparently used to designate a vessel under quarantine in the past, it evolved to denote that the ship's captain considered his ship disease-free and thus ready for boarding and inspection by public health authorities in the hope that quarantine would be lifted. Its past association with quarantine for yellow fever led to the term "Yellow Jack," as it is sometimes referred to in naval lingo.

CONTENTS

FOREWORD

Welcome to this inaugural edition of the *Nebraska Isolation & Quarantine Manual*.

In 2005 the organizations that would eventually comprise Nebraska Medicine opened the Nebraska Biocontainment Unit (NBU), with the support of the Centers for Disease Control and Prevention (CDC). The NBU was the third dedicated patient biocontainment unit to open in the United States. The vision of Dr. Phil Smith, then head of the Division of Infectious Diseases, drove the development of the NBU and was inspired by the recent experiences of the anthrax attacks of 2001, the SARS outbreak of 2002–3, and the 2003 outbreak of monkeypox in the midwestern United States. The 10-bed unit and dedicated supporting facilities were planned carefully, incorporating unique and robust engineering, administrative, and personal protective controls.

Most importantly, the NBU assembled and trained a dedicated and multidisciplinary team of health care professionals and scientists. They collectively researched known best practices, drafted protocols, and practiced repeatedly. Over this time the team became a true family of talented and caring professionals. In 2014 the team's decade-long commitment was tested as the NBU activated in order to care for three patients with Ebola virus disease (EVD) repatriated from West Africa.

Capitalizing on this experience, the UNMC/Nebraska Medicine team joined Emory University and the New York Health and Hospitals Corporation, Bellevue Hospital Center, to found the National Ebola Training and Education Center (NETEC). This federally designated center leads national efforts to improve infection control procedures and practices, as well as isolation and quarantine capabilities, at medical facilities throughout the United States. Through the NETEC, our team is able to share their expertise for best practices and team-based training with hundreds of designated facilities across the nation.

We see the *Nebraska Isolation & Quarantine Manual* as an opportunity to expand our ability to share our experiences and lessons learned with a broader professional audience. We feel strongly that if health care and affiliated professionals become more proficient in the basic principles shared herein, we can improve preparedness for catastrophic infectious disease outbreaks and mitigate their effects, while improving delivery of care overall. At UNMC/Nebraska Medicine, we are committed in our growing efforts to build a safer and healthier nation and global community.

It is an honor to dedicate this manual to our colleague and friend, Dr. Phil Smith, a true, quiet, and unsung hero in every sense of the word. Phil's vision, tireless efforts, compassion, dedicated leadership, and enduring friendship are an inspiration to all of us who care for patients with highly hazardous communicable diseases.

Jeffrey P. Gold
Chancellor, University of Nebraska Medical Center
Chancellor, University of Nebraska at Omaha
Chair, Nebraska Medicine Health System Board

PREFACE

The threat posed by high-consequence infections has become increasingly complex, dangerous, and imminent in our 21st-century environment. Naturally occurring outbreaks such as Ebola, SARS, MERS, and avian influenza have challenged local and regional health care delivery capabilities and impacted economic, social, and political systems. We dodged a bullet when the 2009 H1N1 influenza pandemic turned out to be milder than historic novel flu pandemics, but persisting outbreaks of H7N9 and other avian influenza viruses remind us that the specter of an emerging severe pandemic is ever-present. In addition, rapid advances in biotechnology continue to lower the bar for malevolent use of lethal biological agents. More than ever, our hospitals and health care workers must possess the necessary knowledge and skills to provide effective care for patients infected with highly communicable and highly virulent pathogens while protecting themselves and their families, their health care colleagues, and the public from the spread of infection. This is why I am privileged to introduce the publication of this inaugural edition of the *Nebraska Isolation & Quarantine Manual*.

As the Assistant Secretary for Preparedness and Response (ASPR), I lead an organization that is charged with a singular and critical mission: saving lives and protecting Americans from 21st-century health security threats. On behalf of the Secretary of Health and Human Services (HHS), ASPR leads public health and medical preparedness, response, and recovery for disasters and public health emergencies. Among its many functions, ASPR promotes readiness at the state and local levels by coordinating federal grants and cooperative agreements and carrying out drills and operational exercises. To strengthen domestic response capabilities for high-consequence infectious diseases, HHS/ASPR and the Centers for Disease Control and Prevention (CDC) work with state health departments and the private sector to establish and maintain a nationwide, regional treatment network for Ebola and other highly infectious diseases. In conjunction, HHS awarded funding to establish the National Ebola Training and Education Center (NETEC) to educate and train clinicians to provide safe and supportive care for patients with these diseases. NETEC is a consortium of Emory University, University of Nebraska Medical Center/Nebraska Medicine (UNMC/NM), and New York City Health and Hospitals Corporation/HHC Bellevue Hospital, three US hospitals that treated Ebola patients successfully during the 2014–16 emergency.

As a core member of NETEC and with more than 15 years of history in training, research, and clinical operations for high-consequence infection patient care, I am grateful to our partners at UNMC/NM who continue the tradition of sharing their expertise and helping colleagues around the country meet the challenges of known and emerging infectious disease threats. With the establishment of the Global Center for Health Security at Nebraska, I look forward to their increasing role as both a national and international leader for health system preparedness and response. This manual fills an important gap in civilian biopreparedness, and I hope readers can incorporate its lessons into building more prepared and resilient health care systems and communities.

Robert Kadlec, MD
Assistant Secretary for Preparedness and Response (ASPR)
HHS Office of the Secretary

CONTRIBUTORS

Brenda Ang MBBS MMed MPH
LKC School of Medicine, Singapore
Chapter 11

Elizabeth L. Beam PhD RN
University of Nebraska Medical Center
Chapter 8

Kate C. Boulter RN BAN MPH
Nebraska Medicine
Chapters 9, 20

Christopher K. Brown PhD MPH CPH
Occupational Safety and
Health Administration
Chapter 19

David S. Cates PhD
Nebraska Medicine
Chapter 9

Theodore J. Cieslak MD MPH
University of Nebraska Medical Center
Chapters 1, 4, 15, 16

Wael ElRayes MBBCh PhD FACHE
University of Nebraska Medical Center
Chapter 5

Robert Emery DrPH CHP CIH CBSP
CSP CHMM CPP ARM
The University of Texas Health
Science Center at Houston
Chapter 8

Michael L. Flueckiger MD
Phoenix Air Group
Chapter 18

Shawn G. Gibbs PhD MBA CIH
Indiana University
Chapters 8, 18, 19

Jonathan Grein MD
Cedars-Sinai Medical Center
Chapter 14

Vicki L. Herrera MS
University of Nebraska Medical Center
Chapter 17

Jocelyn J. Herstein MPH PhD
University of Nebraska Medical Center
Chapter 18

Angela L. Hewlett MD MS
University of Nebraska Medical Center
Chapters 1, 7, 9

Selin B. Hoboy BS
Stericycle Inc.
Chapter 19

Jolene M. Horihan RT(R)(M)(ARRT)
Nebraska Medicine
Chapter 9

John P. Horton MD
Emory University
Chapter 16

Peter C. Iwen MS PhD
University of Nebraska Medical Center
Chapter 17

Katelyn C. Jelden MPH
University of Nebraska Medical Center
Chapter 18

Daniel W. Johnson MD
University of Nebraska Medical Center
Chapter 9

Mark G. Kortepeter MD MPH
University of Nebraska Medical Center
Chapters 4, 10, 16

Colleen S. Kraft MD MSc
Emory University
Chapter 22

James V. Lawler MD MPH
University of Nebraska Medical Center
Chapters 2, 5, 8

Aurora B. Le MPH CPH ASP
Indiana University
Chapters 8, 19

Yee-Sin Leo MBBS MMed
FRCP MPH FAMS
National Centre for Infectious
Diseases, Singapore
Chapter 11

Rachel E. Lookadoo JD
University of Nebraska Medical Center
Chapter 3

John J. Lowe PhD
University of Nebraska Medical Center
Chapters 8, 18

Susan L. F. McLellan MD MPH
University of Texas Medical Branch at
Galveston
Chapter 13

Scott J. Patlovich DrPH CIH CBSP
SM(NRCM) CHMM CPH
The University of Texas Health Science
Center at Houston
Chapter 8

Caitlin S. Pedati MD MPH
Iowa Department of Public Health
Chapter 21

Craig A. Piquette MD FACP FCCP
University of Nebraska Medical Center
Chapter 9

George F. Risi MD MSc
Biomedical Advanced Research
and Development Authority
Chapter 12

Elizabeth R. Schnaubelt MD
University of Nebraska Medical Center
Chapter 22

Michelle M. Schwedhelm MSN RN
Nebraska Medicine
Chapters 6, 8

Amanda Strain BSN RN
Nebraska Medicine
Chapter 8

James N. Sullivan MD
University of Nebraska Medical Center
Chapter 9

L. Kate Tyner BSN RN
Nebraska Medicine
Chapter 7

Angela M. Vasa BSN RN
Nebraska Medicine
Chapters 2, 8, 9, 20

Shawn Vasoo MBBS MRCP
D(ABIM) D(ABP)
National Centre for Infectious
Diseases, Singapore
Chapter 11

Michael C. Wadman MD
University of Nebraska Medical Center
Chapter 6

CHAPTER 1

Introduction

THEODORE J. CIESLAK
ANGELA L. HEWLETT

History

The concepts of isolation and quarantine date back thousands of years, with detailed instructions for the assessment and isolation of lepers described in the 13th chapter of the book of Leviticus. In 583, at a council held in Lyon, an edict was issued restricting lepers from freely associating with healthy persons. In the meantime, as the first pandemic of plague swept through Europe, the Byzantine emperor Justinian, in 549, ordered the quarantine of all persons arriving from affected regions. The measure was only partially effective—the plague epidemic arrived despite the quarantine, spread throughout Constantinople and beyond, and ultimately killed at least 13% of the known world's population, putting the final nail in the coffin of the Roman Empire.

When the second global pandemic of plague struck in 1348, Venice established an institutionalized system of quarantine, requiring visiting ships, along with their crews, passengers, and cargoes, to lie at anchor in the Venetian lagoon for 40 days prior to disembarkation. The term "quarantine" (from the Italian *quaranta giorni* [forty days]) derives from the length of this waiting period. In 1374 the duke of Milan added isolation to the repertoire of plague control measures, ordering all victims to be taken to the forest outside the city until they recovered or succumbed.

These measures were also of limited success as the Black Death killed at least 20% of Europe's population. In 1592 a lazaretto (from Lazarus, the leper in Christ's parable and patron saint of those so afflicted), or maritime quarantine station, was established on Malta. While this initial structure was temporary, a permanent facility was constructed in 1643 in order to manage repeated importations of plague and cholera.

In the American colonies, a lazaretto was built on Tybee Island, outside Savannah, Georgia, in 1767, in order to quarantine imported African slaves. By this time, however, quarantine measures had been employed by colonial authorities for at least a century, beginning with a law passed by the New York City General Assembly in 1663. This law, enacted during a smallpox epidemic, prohibited persons arriving from affected areas from entering the city until cleared by sanitary officials.

In 1832 a cholera outbreak killed 30,000 people in Britain, and quarantine efforts shifted toward this disease. New York at that time prohibited ships from approaching within 300 yards of its docks until the absence of cholera aboard could be assured. The failure of this measure (cholera killed an estimated 3,500 in New York that year), as well as the arrival of Asiatic cholera in 1892, prompted the US Congress to pass the National Quarantine Act the following year. This act created, for the first time, a national system of quarantine, with medical standards for the inspection of immigrants, ships, and cargo. At about the same time, President Benjamin Harrison ordered that "no vessel from any foreign port carrying immigrants shall be admitted to . . . the United States until such vessel shall have undergone quarantine detention of twenty days," the shortened duration (from the previous forty) perhaps reflecting a developing understanding of infectious disease incubation periods.

In 1865 King Kamehameha V of Hawaii, facing a leprosy outbreak on the heels of a devastating smallpox epidemic, issued the "act to prevent the spread of leprosy," which, among other things, forced lifelong isolation (on a remote and inaccessible peninsula on the island of Molokai) on thousands of afflicted Hawaiians. In 1892 the Louisiana legislature established a leprosarium at Carville and forcibly moved patients there, again for life. It wasn't until 1969 (on Molokai) and 1970 (in Carville) that residence in a "leper colony" became voluntary. Knowing no other life, a few leprosy patients (now cured) remain at each location to this day.

In 1900 the third global pandemic of plague reached the United States with the death of a Chinese man in San Francisco. The subsequent quarantine imposed on 25,000 people in a 15-block area of the city's Chinese quarter was ruled racist by an intervening court, adding to the burgeoning intense debate over the ethics of quarantine. This debate perhaps reached its zenith in 1907 when Mary Mallon (aka Typhoid Mary) was forcibly quarantined on North Brother Island in New York's East River until 1910, and then again from 1915 until her death in 1938. The ethical conflict over mandatory quarantine was further exacerbated in 1916 when an epidemic of polio struck New York and those wealthy enough to provide a separate bedroom for their sick child could buy their way out of quarantine. Similarly, the incarceration of 30,000 prostitutes during the period 1917–19 in an effort to curb the prevalence of venereal disease has been labeled "the most concerted attack on civil liberties in the name of public health in American history."

By 1945, the availability of penicillin ensured that syphilis and gonorrhea could be cured within a few days, obviating the need for lengthy and controversial quarantine for these diseases. Nonetheless, in Baltimore those few who refused treatment were subject to involuntary hospitalization. Although sanitoria such as the one started by Trudeau in Saranac Lake, New York, in the 1880s already existed for the management of tuberculosis (TB), the first locked TB ward was opened in Seattle in 1949 and served as a model for the construction of similar facilities throughout the United States. The occasional imposition of mandatory isolation orders on infectious, but reluctant, TB patients by state and local public health authorities continues to this day.

In the aftermath of the September 11 terror attacks in 2001 (as well as the subsequent anthrax letter attacks), the Centers for Disease Control and Prevention (CDC) drafted the Model State Emergency Health Powers Act, to be used by states as a template in improving and strengthening their public health response capabilities. Concomitantly, the CDC increased the number of its quarantine stations to 20, located at major international air and sea gateways. It is via these quarantine stations, within the CDC's Division of Global Migration and Quarantine (DGMQ), that persons subject to federal quarantine might first be identified. Whether persons potentially harboring highly hazardous communicable diseases (HHCDs) are identified within the United States or repatriated from abroad (as occurred with most individuals managed during the West Africa Ebola outbreak), public health officials at all levels of government, as well as clinicians, hospital administrators, and emergency planners, will require a working knowledge of isolation and quarantine fundamentals. This book is for them.

Definitions

Isolation, in a clinical context, and as defined by the CDC, refers to the separation of "ill persons who have a communicable disease from those who are healthy." **Quarantine**, on the other hand, is used to "separate and restrict the movement of well persons who may have been exposed to a communicable disease to see if they become ill." The World Health Organization (WHO) broadens these definitions, noting that isolation involves the separation of not only ill or contaminated persons but also "affected baggage, containers, conveyances, goods or postal parcels from others in such a manner as to prevent the spread of infection or contamination," while quarantine refers to the "restriction of activities and/or separation from others of suspect persons who are not ill or of suspect baggage, containers, conveyances or goods" for the same reason.

Restriction of Movement is a term sometimes used in conjunction with both isolation and quarantine, as well as certain travel restrictions and enforced social distancing. **Directed Health Measures**, as defined by the Nebraska Department of Health and Human Services (DHHS) and codified in Nebraska state law, include isolation and quarantine, social distancing, and a number of additional infection control and prevention measures, such as hand and cough hygiene; cleaning, disinfection, and sterilization; decontamination; and the use of personal protective equipment. Other states have their own regulations and definitions.

Isolation can be voluntary or involuntary and may be accomplished in a number of settings. Isolation in the home is a commonly employed public health measure. Most parents are quite familiar with the notion that children with chicken pox and other highly communicable diseases should not return to school or day care until their period of contagion has passed. Among patients requiring outpatient medical care or inpatient hospitalization, isolation is routinely employed in "conventional" clinical settings in the form of a private room coupled with contact or droplet precautions. Such measures, and the diseases warranting their use, are discussed in greater detail in chapter 7. Similarly, patients with TB and a few other diseases transmitted by droplet nuclei (see chapter 14) are typically managed in negatively pressured airborne infection isolation rooms (AIIRs) using airborne precautions when there is a need for hospitalization. Finally, a small number of highly infectious, highly communicable, and highly hazardous infectious diseases (see chapter 4) pose special challenges and generate significant concerns related to employing adequate isolation precautions in a conventional hospital setting. Patients with these diseases, which are described in detail in chapters 10–13, can be considered candidates for management in specialized biocontainment units.

Quarantine can also be voluntary or involuntary and similarly can be managed in a variety of settings. Given that most infectious diseases are not communicable until patients are symptomatic, persons who are deemed reliable by public health authorities can often forego quarantine with instructions to take their temperature frequently and report in if they develop signs or symptoms of disease. When quarantine is required, it can be accomplished within the home in the majority of cases; however, when institutional quarantine is advisable, it is typically imposed by state and local health departments. Various settings may be used, such as unused hospital wards, hotels, and other conventional and comfortable environments. While federal quarantine is expected to remain an infrequent event, changing human behaviors and movement, such as burgeoning migration and ease of global travel, make it likely that exotic and hazardous communicable diseases will occur domestically with increasing frequency. Federal authorities have jurisdiction over travelers arriving from abroad, as well as those engaged in interstate travel and commerce; therefore, we anticipate a concomitant increasing emphasis on the need for a federal quarantine facility. Regardless of whether quarantine is voluntary or mandatory, and whether it is imposed at the local, state, or federal level, recent history demonstrates that serious communicable diseases will continue to emerge and that quarantine and isolation care will be important tools for managing them.

CHAPTER 2

Tiered National System

JAMES V. LAWLER

ANGELA M. VASA

Introduction

The 2014–16 West Africa Ebola virus disease (EVD) outbreak, with resulting domestic importations of EVD cases, revealed that United States health care and public health systems were inadequately prepared to care for patients with highly hazardous communicable disease (HHCD) presenting to hospitals. In response, the federal government worked with state and local health authorities to develop a tiered system of acute care facilities, defined by specific standards, supported by education and training resources, and designed to safely care for future patients with EVD and manage the appearance of other HHCD patients. Currently, this system consists of a network of frontline health care facilities, Ebola assessment hospitals, Ebola treatment centers (ETCs), and ten regional Ebola and other special pathogen treatment centers (RESPTCs), conforming to the ten US regions for preparedness and response defined by the US Department of Health and Human Services (HHS). These facilities are provided with guidance by the National Ebola Training and Education Center (NETEC), the Centers for Disease Control and Prevention (CDC), the HHS Assistant Secretary for Preparedness and Response (ASPR), and public health emergency response elements of the federal government, including CDC Ebola response teams

(CERTs). Collectively, this tiered system, according to an HHS ASPR report, "balances geographic need, considers differences in institutional capabilities, accounts for the potential need to care for a patient with Ebola," and provides the foundation for care of other HHCDs. This chapter describes the current US tiered system, the roles that hospitals and acute care facilities can play, and the resources available to support such entities.

Background and Origin

In September 2014 the West Africa EVD epidemic was already the largest known outbreak of EVD in history and had resulted in thousands of deaths in West Africa. Amid rising concerns about the potential for imported cases of EVD, several hospitals in the United States and Europe treated repatriated, infected relief workers—but in specialized units that had trained specifically for management of HHCDs. Then, on September 30, the first unplanned case of EVD imported to the United States was admitted to a Dallas hospital. By the time the patient died in the hospital eight days later, two staff nurses were infected with EVD, contradicting previous claims that standard hospital infection prevention and control training and procedures should prove adequate to prevent nosocomial transmission. These events triggered a scramble among hospitals and the public health authorities to prepare the US health system to manage the potential influx of new cases.

By late October 2014, EVD treatment experts along with federal, state, and local health authorities agreed that EVD patients in the United States should be funneled to referral centers that had appropriate training and infrastructure to safely manage such infections. Out of necessity, health authorities began to take a regional and tiered approach to designating and training hospitals to serve in that role. The CDC developed and implemented training in hospitals in perceived highest-risk locations. In early December 2014 CDC designated 35 hospitals as ETCs that had been trained and inspected by CERTs and had developed interim guidance with additional training materials for hospitals occupying a frontline role in the tiered system. In addition, training teams and new training materials on a variety of media (including Apple's iTunes

University) were developed and pushed out by expert groups such as the Nebraska Biocontainment Unit at Nebraska Medicine (NM)/University of Nebraska Medical Center (UNMC) in order to supplement activities from CDC and other official government sources. Using $260 million in 2015 Ebola supplemental funds and congressional authorization, the CDC and ASPR Hospital Preparedness Program (HPP) developed a concept for a regional treatment network for EVD by August 2015 and had launched additional training and support efforts to realize that goal.

US Regional Treatment System for EVD

The tiered, regional system concept recognizes that the care of patients with EVD (and other HHCDs) is hazardous, highly complex, and best implemented by clinical care teams with specific technical expertise and technological and logistical systems. However, it also acknowledges the reality that these patients can present to any hospital at any time. Therefore, all facilities must be prepared to identify, isolate, and provide initial clinical management for patients under investigation (PUIs) until safe transport can be arranged to a more capable hospital. While guidance exists for out-patient clinics and other health care facilities regarding the identification and initial management of a PUI, the tiered system is designed to encompass specifically acute care facilities: hospitals and urgent care facilities specializing in treatment of acutely ill patients that will likely be the point of entry and initial point of significant clinical intervention for PUI presenting to the health care system. While it is a national system, designation of hospital roles and coordination of regional networks occur among partners within the region to ensure it serves the specific local need.

To achieve a robust capability, the US system encourages acute health care facilities and hospitals to occupy one of four roles:

1. Regional Ebola and other special pathogen treatment center (one for each of the ten HHS regions)

2. Ebola treatment center (state or jurisdiction)

3. Ebola assessment hospital

4. Frontline health care facility

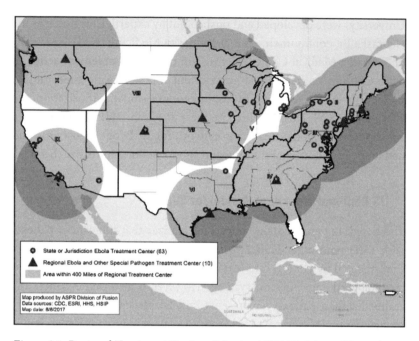

Figure 2.1. Regional Treatment Centers (Map by ASPR Division of Fusion)

Frontline facility and assessment hospital roles emphasize early identification and the ability to safely and effectively care for EVD patients on a temporary basis until transportation is arranged to higher-tier facilities. Frontline facilities should have sufficient staffing and supplies to provide care to an EVD patient for 12–24 hours prior to transfer. Assessment hospitals should be prepared to manage patients for up to 96 hours. Both ETCs and RESPTCs should be capable of providing definitive care and sustained management for patients with EVD or other HHCDs, although the RESPTCs are preferred as they should possess more robust capacity. CDC guidance and description of capabilities for the various levels is summarized in Table 2.1 and located at the CDC's website: https://www.cdc.gov/vhf/ebola/healthcare-us /preparing/hospitals.html.

As we write this chapter, health authorities have designated more than 4,800 frontline health care facilities and more than 200 Ebola assessment hospitals. Sixty-three hospitals are considered ETCs, and the 10 RESPTCs are positioned so that a significant majority of the United States is located within 400 miles of an RESPTC. A map of treatment centers is contained in Figure 2.1.

Support for Regional Treatment Network Facilities

A number of resources exist to support facilities with respect to education and training in preparedness, just-in-time training, subject matter expertise, or operational assistance in response activities. The centerpiece of support is NETEC, a consortium of three academic medical centers: Emory University Medical Center, Nebraska Medicine/ University of Nebraska Medical Center, and New York City Hospitals/ Bellevue Medical Center, which successfully managed EVD patients during the 2014–16 epidemic. CDC and ASPR established NETEC in parallel with the tiered regional network concept with the purpose of serving as the hub for developing and delivering education and training for EVD care. Among its functions, NETEC develops a suite of exercise templates addressing EVD care to be used by coalitions and individual health care facilities, provides readiness consultations for all designated facilities to assess preparedness efforts, provides real-time technical assistance, and supports a special pathogen clinical research infrastructure in the United States. Through NETEC, institutions can find a diverse collection of resources to assist in their efforts to advance readiness for HHCDs, accessible at https://netec.org/.

In addition to NETEC, CDC and ASPR provide guidance and education tailored for all tiers. CDC's website contains information regarding hospital preparedness and the care of PUIs and confirmed EVD patients (see the link above). The website links to specific information for each tier of the network as well as various aspects of identification, isolation, and management of cases. ASPR's Technical Resources, Assistance Center, and Information Exchange (TRACIE) is a resource developed for a wide range of federal and nonfederal entities involved in preparedness and response for public health emergencies. The TRACIE website is accessible at https://asprtracie.hhs.gov. The website provides a portal to technical and guidance documents, subject matter expertise

Table 2.1 Health Care Facility Guidance by Tier

Tier	Capability	Planned and prepared duration of care
Regional Ebola and other special pathogen treatment center (RESPTC)	• Receive and isolate up to 2 patients with EVD within 8 hours of notification • Provide clinical care for EVD patients for duration of illness using appropriate infection prevention and control (IPC) practice • Treat pediatric cases of EVD and other HHCD • Isolate and care for up to 10 patients with pathogen infections transmitted by respiratory/aerosol route • Safely manage hazardous waste from EVD patients	Duration of illness–PPE on hand for 7 days' operation
Ebola treatment center (ETC)	• Receive and isolate a patient with confirmed EVD • Provide clinical care for EVD patient for duration of illness • Coordinate disposal of Category A waste with commercial vendor or appropriate entity • Work with state, local, and regional partners to coordinate interfacility transfer of patient with EVD	Duration of illness–PPE on hand for 7 days' operation
Regional Ebola and other special pathogen treatment center (RESPTC)	• Receive and isolate up to 2 patients with EVD within 8 hours of notification • Provide clinical care for EVD patients for duration of illness using appropriate infection prevention and control (IPC) practice • Treat pediatric cases of EVD and other HHCD • Isolate and care for up to 10 patients with pathogen infections transmitted by respiratory/aerosol route • Safely manage hazardous waste from EVD patients	Duration of illness–PPE on hand for 7 days' operation

Table 2.1 Health Care Facility Guidance by Tier (continued)

Tier	Capability	Planned and prepared duration of care
Ebola treatment center (ETC)	• Receive and isolate a patient with confirmed EVD • Provide clinical care for EVD patient for duration of illness • Coordinate disposal of Category A waste with commercial vendor or appropriate entity • Work with state, local, and regional partners to coordinate interfacility transfer of patient with EVD	Duration of illness–PPE on hand for 7 days' operation
Ebola assessment hospital	• Receive and isolate a PUI • Provide immediate laboratory evaluation and arrange for Ebola diagnostic testing • Provide necessary medical treatment using appropriate IPC, including care for alternative diagnoses • Coordinate disposal of Category A waste with commercial vendor or appropriate entity • Work with state, local, and regional partners to coordinate transfer of patient to ETC or RSPTC	96 hours
Frontline health care facility	• Rapidly identify and isolate a PUI • Notify local personnel and appropriate public health authorities to arrange transfer • Provide necessary medical treatment using appropriate IPC	12–24 hours

and assistance with answering questions on specific preparedness or response topics, and discussion boards for peer-to-peer information exchange. The TRACIE assistance center can be accessed online or through a toll-free number (1-844-5-TRACIE) but is only staffed during working hours and is not an appropriate resource for acute needs related to response.

In the event of an actual PUI or confirmed Ebola patient, facilities can reach out to several real-time resources. Local and state public health authorities should always be the first point of contact and should be made aware of any other outreach. The CDC Emergency Operations Center (EOC) hotline is available 24/7 as a single point of contact to access CDC subject matter experts. The CDC EOC watch officer is available at 770-488-7100. If on-site assistance is required, a CDC Ebola Response Team (CERT) can deploy to provide direct support to hospitals. NETEC also provides on-call support for technical assistance and advice. Individual hospitals can access NETEC subject matter experts either by contacting their state health department or through the CDC EOC, who have direct access to the NETEC emergency consultation phone line.

Regional Network and HHCDs Other Than Ebola

Although the regional treatment system was conceived to address EVD and funded by appropriations specifically tied to the response to the 2014–16 Ebola crisis, ASPR and CDC acknowledge that the network can and should be used to address a myriad of HHCD threats requiring specialized care and IPC. Guidance specifically calls for RESPTCs to have capability to manage airborne respiratory pathogens, and much of the training and exercised capabilities established under the tiered system should be directly transferrable to management of other HHCDs requiring enhanced contact, droplet, or airborne precautions. Under the ASPR HPP Ebola Preparedness Measures released in 2017, designated facilities conducting exercises with "other special pathogens" were allowed to include these efforts in the reporting requirements to meet specified metrics. ETCs and assessment hospitals must conduct, at a minimum, annual exercises, and RESPTCs must complete quarterly exercises including no-notice components. RESPTCs are also required to conduct quarterly training for all rostered staff including IPC practices and PPE donning and doffing.

In order to support the evolution from EVD-centric preparedness efforts, NETEC, in collaboration with ASPR and CDC, have developed exercise templates that are customizable for different HHCDs of concern and map directly to the ASPR HPP Ebola Preparedness metrics, which enable all tiered facilities to more effectively plan and execute required exercises. In addition, NETEC readiness consultations now include considerations related to airborne respiratory pathogens for facilities and subject matters on site to address during the consultation.

Conclusion

The advent of the tiered regional system for care of EVD and other HHCD patients significantly advanced the ability of the US health care system to identify, isolate, treat, and transport these patients in a way that protects health care workers and others. This initiative, along with the implementation of NETEC working alongside federal agencies, ultimately strengthens the nation's health care and public health systems for the next emerging infectious disease threat. Health care facilities should work with local and state public health authorities and their local health care coalition to determine the appropriate tier they should occupy and coordinate training and exercise plans to integrate fully within their region's network. Guidance and training resources for each tier are available through CDC and NETEC, among others. As the threat of novel emerging infections continues to grow, this system should serve as a cornerstone for future efforts to mitigate the impact of these significant and dangerous events.

CHAPTER 3

Legal Considerations

RACHEL E. LOOKADOO

When dealing with issues of isolation and quarantine, legal considerations may be forgotten in the midst of clinical concerns. However, as
there are numerous laws and regulations that apply to quarantine matters, these issues must be considered. Additionally, while holding an individual under quarantine, it is critical to ensure that their rights are
maintained and respected. This chapter reviews the various laws that
govern quarantine matters in the United States and outlines the rights of
individuals being quarantined.

Jurisdiction

In the United States, issues of isolation and quarantine typically fall
under a state's jurisdiction. However, state laws are not the only laws
governing these types of issues. Federal laws and regulations have been
issued that delineate the circumstances under which federal quarantine
orders may be authorized. Additionally, as a member state of the World
Health Organization (WHO), the United States must also follow the requirements of the International Health Regulations (IHRs). This section
breaks down the requirements of each jurisdiction and when each set of
laws and regulations applies.

In 2005, in response to the 2003 severe acute respiratory syndrome (SARS) outbreak, the World Health Assembly approved the revised IHRs. The IHRs are an international treaty agreed upon by 196 countries, including all of the member states of the WHO. As one of these member states, the United States has agreed to follow these regulations. The goal of the IHRs is to prevent the international spread of disease and provide a public health response to such an event. Rather than being limited to any specific disease, the IHRs are general and apply to any "illness or medical condition, irrespective of origin or source, which presents, or could present, significant harm to humans." In addition to establishing public health surveillance and response standards, the IHRs also contain a notice requirement. Under these regulations, if an event occurs that is determined to be a Public Health Emergency of International Concern (PHEIC), then the country involved must notify the WHO within 24 hours. In the United States, all PHEIC notifications are made by the US IHR National Focal Point (NFP), within the office of the Assistant Secretary for Preparedness and Response (ASPR) within the Department of Health and Human Services (HHS). State and local health departments are responsible for maintaining surveillance and reporting nationally notifiable diseases/conditions to the federal government. By notifying the state and local health departments of notifiable diseases, hospitals, health care facilities, and quarantine centers are helping ensure that any necessary reporting will occur.

FEDERAL QUARANTINE

The federal government has a significant interest in maintaining the health and well-being of US citizens. In furtherance of that interest, the federal government has the authority to take steps to prevent the transmission, introduction, or spread of communicable diseases through statutory and regulatory mandates. Additionally, executive orders are issued to specify those diseases that might be considered for quarantine. In carrying out these laws, regulations, and orders, different operational mechanisms are used, including federal quarantine stations.

The federal laws governing quarantine and isolation are found in the

Public Health Service (PHS) Act (42 United States Code 264). Enacted in 1944, this law created the federal government's authority to isolate and quarantine individuals. The statute calls for the secretary of HHS to create regulations to prevent the introduction, transmission, or spread of communicable diseases from foreign countries into the United States, or from one state into another. These statutorily mandated regulations only apply to communicable diseases specified by the president through executive orders.

The statute also differentiates the requirements for detaining or examining foreign or interstate travelers. For interstate travelers, any individual who is reasonably believed to be infected with a communicable disease may be apprehended or examined if the following two conditions are met. First, the disease must be in a qualifying stage, which is defined as being either in a precommunicable (if the disease would be likely to cause a public health emergency if transmitted to other individuals) or communicable stage. Second, the individual believed to be infected must be either moving from one state to another, or be "a probable source of infection to individuals who, while infected with such disease in a qualifying stage, will be moving from a state to another state." If those requirements are met, then the individual may be examined and, if found to be infected, detained for such a time and in such a manner as is reasonably necessary. For foreign travelers, the qualifying stage and interstate travel requirements do not need to be met in order to apprehend, detain, examine, or conditionally release an individual. This statute also states that while state law will generally govern matters of quarantine, if there is a conflict between state and federal law, the federal law will preempt the state law.

To help enforce the PHS Act, HHS created regulations that give the Centers for Disease Control and Prevention (CDC) the authority to carry out the federal government's quarantine powers. These regulations apply only to federal quarantine orders, not state or local quarantine orders. The regulations were most recently updated in January 2017 to include revisions based on the response to the 2014 Ebola outbreak.

The CDC regulations are split into two parts: part 70 covers interstate introduction, transmission, and spread of communicable disease, and part 71 covers foreign introduction, transmission, and spread of communicable disease. Both parts contain regulations relating to the manner in which the CDC can monitor travelers for disease on airlines, in airports, and at other ports of entry. The regulations also require that an individual under a federal isolation or quarantine order may not be permitted to travel between states without a travel permit issued by the CDC. This requirement is of note because it can also apply to state and local quarantine orders, if the state or local authority with jurisdiction requests federal assistance. If an individual requests a travel permit and is denied, then he or she may appeal the decision to the CDC director.

According to the regulations, in order to isolate or quarantine someone, there must be a reasonable belief based on specific facts that would lead a public health officer to conclude that the individual has been exposed to a communicable disease and is, or may be, harboring the infectious agent of that disease in his or her body. In order to determine those facts, the individual in question must undergo a medical exam. On the issuance of a federal quarantine or isolation order, written notice must be given to the quarantined individual informing them of their rights. The individual must also be informed that an automatic reassessment of the quarantine order will occur within 72 hours of being served the order. If, as a result of the reassessment, a determination is made for more detention time, then the individual can request an additional review.

As referenced above, the CDC may apprehend, detain, and examine individuals to prevent the spread and transmission of certain communicable diseases. These diseases are specified by the president through executive orders. Since the passing of the PHS Act in 1944, seven such executive orders have been issued. According to Executive Order 13295 and its amendments, the following diseases justify the use of federal quarantine and isolation measures:

- Cholera;
- Diphtheria;
- Infectious tuberculosis;
- Plague;
- Smallpox;
- Yellow fever;

Nebraska Isolation & Quarantine Manual

- Viral hemorrhagic fevers (Lassa, Marburg, Ebola, Crimean-Congo, South American, and others not yet isolated or named);

- Severe acute respiratory syndromes (e.g., SARS and Middle East respiratory syndrome [MERS]), diseases associated with fever and signs and symptoms of pneumonia or other respiratory illness, capable of being transmitted from person to person, and causing, or having the potential to cause, a pandemic, or, on infection, are highly likely to cause mortality or serious morbidity if not properly controlled; and

- Influenza caused by novel or reemergent influenza viruses that are causing, or have the potential to cause, a pandemic.

This list only applies to *federal* isolation and quarantine measures, not *state* measures. States are not limited by this list and can create their own list of diseases that call for isolation or quarantine.

As part of the CDC's quarantine authority, federal quarantine stations were created across the United States to serve as barriers to the introduction of communicable diseases into the country. There are twenty such quarantine stations located at major ports of entry and land-border crossings where the majority of international travelers arrive. If an individual is reported to be ill on an international flight or other form of travel into the United States, then a CDC health officer at the quarantine station will determine whether that individual may enter the United States. Additionally, CDC health officers inspect cargo and animals/products at the quarantine stations to ensure that any threats or vectors of communicable diseases do not enter the country.

STATE AND LOCAL QUARANTINE

Since the passing of federal quarantine laws, federal quarantine powers have very rarely been invoked. As the federal rules apply only to communicable disease incidents crossing international or state borders, state and local laws govern most situations of isolation and/or quarantine. States have the power to govern quarantine through the broad police powers given to the states through the Tenth Amendment to the US Constitution. These police powers give states the authority to protect the health and welfare of the public, including the authority to take precautions such as quarantine.

Quarantine laws vary significantly among states, particularly in regard to the specific rights that are enumerated for individuals being quarantined. For example, only 14 states allow quarantined individuals to choose their own health care provider. Additionally, states differ in whether they place quarantine powers with the state or local health departments. In the State of Nebraska, both the state department of health and human services and the local public health departments have the authority to issue quarantine orders.

Since state laws can vary considerably, please be sure to check with your state or local public health department to determine what the laws are in your jurisdiction.

Patient and Personal Rights

While both federal and state governments have broad authority to prevent the spread of communicable diseases, individuals' constitutional rights must still be upheld and protected. One of the most critical of these rights is an individual's right to due process. Under the Fifth and Fourteenth Amendments, federal and state governments are prohibited from depriving a citizen of "life, liberty, or property, without due process of law." In order to justify depriving an individual's liberty by placing them in quarantine, the government must show a compelling interest in protecting the public health by preventing the spread of disease. Also under these amendments, individuals are given equal protection rights that, for quarantine purposes, mean that any quarantine or isolation measures must be nondiscriminatory in their scope and application.

RIGHT TO COUNSEL

Under the CDC regulations, an individual who is subject to a federal order for quarantine, isolation, or conditional release may request a medical review of the order. This review is intended to determine whether the CDC has a reasonable belief that the individual is infected with quarantinable communicable disease. At this review, the quarantined individual is entitled to be represented by an advocate, such as an attorney. In the event that the individual is indigent, meaning their annual family income is below 200% of the applicable poverty guidelines, then the government will appoint an attorney at its expense to represent the individual.

For state quarantine orders, an individual's right to counsel varies by state. As of this writing, only 23 states have explicitly granted a right to counsel for quarantined individuals. As the right to counsel is considered a basic due process right under the Constitution, it is a best practice to ensure that quarantined individuals have a right to an attorney. If you are unsure as to what your local state laws may be regarding this issue, please consult with your state or local health department.

RIGHT TO A HABEAS PETITION

When an individual is detained by the government, a petition for a writ of habeas corpus may be granted so that the individual may seek relief from their detention. The right to a habeas petition is guaranteed through the due process clause of the Fifth Amendment. While these types of petitions are predominantly used in criminal detention situations, they are also relevant in matters of quarantine. If a petition for a writ of habeas corpus is granted, then a hearing is held to determine whether there is sufficient legal cause to justify the individual's detention. The federal regulations explicitly state that nothing in the quarantine order can interfere with an individual's constitutional right to judicial review, meaning the right to a habeas petition. However, there is no consistent procedure for individuals seeking a writ of habeas corpus for state quarantine orders. Processes vary across states, with some states specifically addressing habeas rights, and other states not addressing them at all. To determine the process for seeking a petition for a writ of habeas corpus in your state, consult your state laws and regulations.

RIGHT TO FOOD, MEDICINE, AND OTHER NECESSITIES

Under the CDC regulations, an individual who has been apprehended or held in quarantine or isolation will be provided adequate food and water, appropriate accommodation, appropriate medical treatment, and means of necessary communication. These provisions apply only to federal quarantine orders.

As with the other personal rights of quarantined individuals, state law varies regarding these provisions. While some states provide all medical care, lodging, and food, some states require individuals to pay for their own food, accommodations, and medical care. If you are unsure as to how your state handles these provisions, please consult your state laws and regulations.

Additionally, there is no provision for a right to compensation under the regulations associated with federal quarantine orders. In the case of state and local quarantine orders, the laws vary. Only 20% of states provide employment protection for individuals who cannot work while under quarantine or isolation. Please check your local or state laws to determine whether quarantined individuals are compensated in your jurisdiction.

Practical Guidance

When dealing with an isolation or quarantine situation, it is important to keep in mind that every situation is different and that each state handles things differently. As federal quarantine orders have rarely been issued in the past, it is most likely that any quarantine order you face will be coming from a state or local level. With that in mind, ensure that you can readily access correct and up-to-date contact information for your local public health department and state health department. Those entities will be best able to give you clarifying information regarding your specific jurisdiction's rules and processes. If it is determined that the situation has escalated to the point that it meets the CDC statutory standards for federal quarantine, contact the CDC quarantine station for your jurisdiction. A map of the quarantine stations and their contact information can be found at https://www.cdc.gov/quarantine /quarantinestationcontactlistfull.html.

CHAPTER 4

Pathogens of Concern

THEODORE J. CIESLAK
MARK G. KORTEPETER

Contagious infectious pathogens spread person to person by a variety of means, which impact their ability to be transmitted within health care settings. Widespread consensus exists regarding the specific infectious diseases requiring contact, droplet, and airborne precautions in conventional health care settings. These, as well as the specific infection control modalities utilized for implementing the precautions, are catalogued in the CDC's Healthcare Infection Control Practice Advisory Committee's (HICPAC) publication, *2007 Guideline for Isolation Precautions: Preventing Transmission of Infectious Agents in Healthcare Settings*, and are discussed briefly in chapter 7 of this manual.

On the other hand, no universally accepted list of diseases warranting care in a high-level containment care (HLCC) unit currently exists, although there have been recent attempts to create such a list. While all of the diseases proposed for care in these specialized units have been managed successfully in conventional settings, the converse is also true. Each of the highly hazardous diseases under consideration has also been managed unsuccessfully in conventional settings, and HLCC can provide an extra and important margin of safety.

Even if HLCC is preferable to care under "conventional" isolation in certain circumstances, such care has several drawbacks. First, HLCC capacity is limited. Only a few dozen HLCC beds exist within the United States, scattered across a handful of facilities. Second, it is extraordinarily costly in terms of financial and human resources. Third, in many cases, it limits visitation by family members, which can be traumatizing for both the patient and family members. Finally, in some cases, it may be counterproductive with respect to safety. Caregivers require extensive and repeated training to reach a level of proficiency in such an environment. They must spend long hours in cumbersome personal protective equipment (PPE), with diminished tactile, visual, and auditory acuity, prone to fatigue-driven mistakes, while the PPE is at risk of snagging on, and upsetting, medical equipment.

Although each care facility has the flexibility to make decisions that optimize safety, for the reasons noted above, we believe that it is prudent to limit admissions to HLCC units to those diseases that meet several specific criteria: diseases should be highly infectious, highly communicable, and highly hazardous. While myriad infectious diseases fulfill at least one of these criteria, few fulfill all three. For example, Q fever (caused by infection with *Coxiella burnetii*) is extraordinarily infectious, with an ID_{50} of as little as a single organism. Likewise, for brucellosis, caused by various species of *Brucella*, the ID_{50} is probably fewer than 10 organisms. Yet neither of these diseases is communicable from person to person. It might also be argued that neither are particularly hazardous, if recognized and treated appropriately. Diseases such as mumps and norovirus-induced gastroenteritis, while perhaps not quite as infectious as Q fever and brucellosis, ARE very communicable, but still not particularly hazardous. Finally, anthrax (caused by *Bacillus anthracis*) is highly hazardous, as demonstrated by the deaths resulting from the 2001 Amerithrax terror attacks, but it is not particularly infectious (the LD_{50} for humans is estimated to be ~8,000–40,000 spores) and is not communicable. In other words, persons exposed to a primary aerosol (as in a terror attack) are at risk of developing anthrax, but health care workers caring for ill victims are not. Botulism deserves special mention. The causative bacteria, *Clostridium botulinum*, produces an intoxication rather than an infection (except in the case of wound botulism), after exposure to a toxin produced by the organism. As such, it, too, is not contagious. Although it is certainly hazardous, without a risk of spread, it would not warrant isolation.

Some infectious diseases fulfill two criteria. Rubella is both highly infectious (ID_{50} = 10–60 virions) and highly communicable, but it isn't particularly hazardous, except to a developing fetus. Similarly, tularemia is highly infectious (ID_{50} = 10 organisms) and highly hazardous (the mortality rate associated with pneumonic tularemia is as high as 30%), but it isn't communicable. Again, there would be no need to manage such diseases under HLCC conditions.

With certain infections, the ID_{50} isn't well established, and infectivity is probably the least important of the three criteria. This is evident when one considers that billions of viral particles may be expelled when infected individuals cough or sneeze, depending on the disease. In this regard, Nipah virus may not be as infectious as some pathogens, but it is communicable and highly hazardous. Consequently, until more is understood about the potential for spread in the nosocomial environment with this pathogen, we would recommend that patients with Nipah virus disease be managed in an HLCC unit when such an asset is available. Finally, there are several diseases that fulfill all three criteria where little controversy exists. Ebola and some other viral hemorrhagic fever (VHF) viruses are highly infectious (ID_{50} as few as one virion), highly communicable, and clearly highly hazardous (with a historical mortality rate of 50–90%). With the VHFs, the environment has a significant impact on how efficiently they spread, because they require close contact with blood and other body fluids. This makes the household and health care settings particularly dangerous. A limited number of severe acute respiratory diseases, such as SARS, MERS, and perhaps certain forms of influenza (caused by avian, prepandemic, and other novel strains) also appear to fulfill these three criteria, as does smallpox. Monkeypox deserves special mention here. Although there were no fatal cases among the 47 that occurred in the American Midwest in 2003, the clinical and virologic similarities between monkeypox and smallpox, coupled with the grave public health implications of even a single case of smallpox, lead us to advocate that a potential monkeypox case should prompt HLCC admission at least until smallpox can be definitively excluded. These concepts are depicted graphically in figure 4.1.

After considering a disease's infectivity, communicability, and hazard, one can apply a fourth criterion: countermeasure availability. For example, polio is certainly highly infectious, highly communicable, and can be quite hazardous, resulting in permanent paralysis in a minority of patients (although the majority of polio victims suffer only mild nonparalytic disease). Nonetheless, very effective vaccines exist, and health care workers, as well as other contacts, can be protected via immunization. Therefore, vaccination of health care workers, coupled with conventional contact isolation procedures, guards adequately against polio transmission and obviates the need for HLCC. Measles provides another example: it is perhaps the most communicable disease known (with a reproduction number [R_0] of 12–18), and measles is also highly infectious. Moreover, despite its reputation as a "routine" childhood exanthem until a few decades ago, measles can be devastating in the setting of vitamin A deficiency. In the developing world, 200,000 children still die each year as a result of measles or its complications. Again, however, an effective vaccine prevents measles; persons with this disease who require hospitalization can thus be managed in an airborne infection isolation room (AIIR) with airborne precautions, after ensuring that caregivers and other contacts are adequately immunized.

The availability of antibiotics obviates the need for HLCC admission of almost any person with a bacterial disease, as patients harboring these are typically rendered noncontagious very quickly. In rare circumstances, if prolonged bacterial shedding may occur despite antibiotic therapy (glanders, as a possible example), caregivers might be given prophylactic antibiotics to supplement their reliance on proper PPE and other infection control methodologies. A few exceptions to this general rule deserve mention, however. Pneumonic plague, caused by the gram-negative coccobacillus *Yersinia pestis*, is so rapidly progressive, with death often occurring within 24 hours after symptom onset, and antibiotic treatment futile if delayed until after pulmonary symptom onset, that patients with pneumonic plague could reasonably be considered candidates for management in an HLCC unit. Finally, extensively drug-resistant strains of *Mycobacterium tuberculosis* (XDR-TB) may be untreatable using currently available antituberculous therapy regimens. While much TB care can be provided without resorting to hospitalization, TB is highly infectious, highly communicable, and quite hazardous. Some experts might thus advocate for managing XDR-TB patients requiring hospitalization in an HLCC setting.

While we have discussed specific diseases that might warrant management in an HLCC environment, we acknowledge that no list will remain static. The future development of new countermeasures may remove some diseases from this list. For example, recent success with a vesicular stomatitis virus-vectored Ebola vaccine in ring vaccination trials holds promise that patients with EVD may someday be adequately cared for in conventional settings by immunized health care workers. Similarly, a licensed vaccine against Junin virus is employed in Argentina. Should Argentinian hemorrhagic fever (AHF), which is caused by the virus, ever become a problem in the United States and the vaccine subsequently be licensed here, this disease may drop off our list of those requiring HLCC. Conversely, dozens of new diseases emerge each year. While most will be controlled utilizing routine infection control practices, inevitably some will prove particularly challenging, with high infectivity, high communicability, and high hazard. We thus allow that the periodic new "Andromeda Strains" will be added to the list of HLCC pathogens in the future.

Finally, we acknowledge that decisions such as who to admit to an HLCC unit may not always be made based on medical aspects alone. The HLCC unit protects at least six groups of individuals. First and foremost, it protects the patient by offering care in a robustly equipped, self-contained unit staffed by selected individuals with extensive expertise in critical care and infectious diseases. Second, it protects the health care worker. Third, it protects other patients from the threat of contagion in the nosocomial environment. Fourth, it protects families by removing difficult decisions about visitation (which is typically not permitted in HLCC units). Fifth, it protects the laboratory worker who may be required to handle specimens containing some of the world's most dangerous pathogens. Finally, it protects the community by offering an additional level of assurance. It is related to this sixth reason that political, media-driven, and public perception–related concerns may, in the future, drive decisions regarding HLCC unit admission, even in cases where the disease in question might not otherwise warrant such. We allow for this possibility.

Taking all of these factors into account, we can assemble a short list (table 4.1) of those conditions that might lead one to consider HLCC

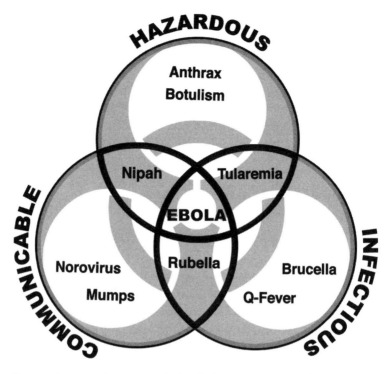

Figure 4.1. Venn Diagram Depicting the Three Factors Used in Determining Whether a Pathogen Warrants Management in an HLCC Unit (Courtesy of Jason Noble)

care. The viral hemorrhagic fevers merit additional clarification. While the viruses that cause these diseases belong to four taxonomic families (much more detailed discussion is provided in chapter 10), the flaviviral VHFs, such as yellow fever and dengue, are not transmissible from person to person, instead requiring an arthropod vector. In addition, VHF can be caused by hantaviruses (within the family *Bunyaviridae*), but these viruses are typically acquired as a result of exposure to rodent excreta rather than person-to-person spread. Therefore, we have omitted those diseases from the group of VHFs that would warrant HLCC care. Each of the remaining VHFs, as well as the other diseases listed in the table, is discussed in detail later in this text (chapters 10–13).

Table 4.1. Diseases That Warrant Consideration for HLCC Care

Viral hemorrhagic fevers	Ebola and Marburg Lassa and Lujo New world arenaviruses Crimean-Congo hemorrhagic fever (CCHF)
Severe respiratory syndromes	SARS and MERS Novel, avian, prepandemic influenza
Orthopoxvirus infections	Smallpox and monkeypox
Henipavirus infections	Nipah and Hendra
Bacterial diseases	Pneumonic plague XDR-TB
Emerging infectious diseases	New diseases that are seemingly highly infectious, contagious, and hazardous
Diseases that provoke an unusual degree of public concern	

CHAPTER 5

Quarantine Unit Operations

WAEL ELRAYES
JAMES V. LAWLER

Quarantine can serve as an integral part of the overall strategy to limit the spread of communicable infections. As the rate of global emerging infectious diseases accelerates and more than 110 million international travelers arrive in the United States each year, it becomes increasingly important for public health authorities to have necessary tools to contain such outbreaks. Traditionally, quarantine is fulfilled in homes, since these persons theoretically are not ill and not contagious. In some circumstances, however, clinical rationale or political considerations support the concept of a dedicated quarantine unit. During the 2014–16 Ebola virus disease (EVD) outbreak, some US public health authorities and the Department of Defense used designated quarantine facilities for persons returning from affected countries. This chapter provides a brief overview of national quarantine systems and considerations around establishing and operating dedicated quarantine units in the United States. In general, quarantine authorities and their implementation are reserved for state and local government. National quarantine authorities do exist to address transborder and interstate spread of disease, however. A more thorough discussion of legal authorities and considerations is contained in chapter 3. The Division of Global Migration and Quarantine (DGMQ) within the Centers for Disease Control and Prevention (CDC) oversees federal quarantine decisions and partners with airport, seaport, and border crossing authorities to limit the introduction of communi-

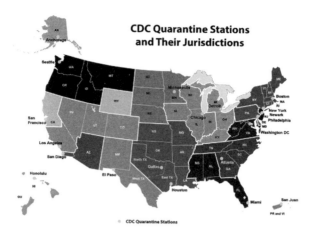

Figure 5.1. Federal Quarantine Stations (Map by CDC)

cable diseases into the United States. DGMQ staffs quarantine stations at 20 major international travel ports of entry. These, in turn, oversee an additional 300 or so airports and border crossing points (Figure 5.1), and serve as frontline locations at which to assess incoming travelers (US and non-US citizens) who may be identified as being ill on their way into the United States. These facilities, which are authorized under 42 CFR, parts 70/71, serve a triage function and screen ill passengers arriving into the United States, ensuring that those in need of care are referred to appropriate facilities. Individuals who are identified as posing a communicable risk are evaluated prior to release. These stations do not perform long-term quarantine, but instead may retain prospective patients for medical evaluation and make a determination as to whether the individual needs quarantine. Individuals can then be referred to local or state health authorities, who can provide definitive quarantine for defined periods of time, depending on the suspected illness. If needed, the quarantine stations are backed up by US Customs and Border Protection and US Coast Guard officers, who have the authority to enforce quarantine orders.

In 2016 the office of the Assistant Secretary for Preparedness and Response (ASPR) provided funding to the University of Nebraska Medical Center (UNMC) and Nebraska Medicine (NM) in Omaha to develop a dedicated federal quarantine facility, known as the National Quarantine Unit (NQU). The mission of the NQU is to enhance the US health security and quarantine capabilities by providing quarantine services to federal, state, and local authorities as well as private entities and individuals, in specially designed quarantine spaces in a manner that enhances health and national security and fulfills quarantine needs within the health care continuum.

Quarantine Activities and Services

Quarantine represents a point on the broad health security continuum, although quarantine is not considered "health care" in the traditional sense, and "persons under quarantine" are not considered patients. Unlike most other points and levels of health care services, it fulfills a very specific purpose and applies to healthy individuals with a "pre-identified" duration of stay. This duration is often guided by international and national health regulations and depends primarily on the disease or condition affecting the quarantined individuals.

Quarantine operations should focus on two goals: minimizing the risk of disease transmission to susceptible members of the community, and providing a safe, secure, healthy, and controlled environment for the person(s) in quarantine. Because most highly dangerous communicable diseases are not transmissible prior to onset of symptoms, the former goal can be achieved through a variety of strategies. Facilities can employ "loose" quarantine standards, as many did during the 2014–16 Ebola outbreak, where quarantined individuals are allowed limited access outside of the secure quarantine area, generally with limits to avoid crowds and busy public spaces. Some cases with high-risk exposures, security threats, or flight risk may warrant more strict quarantine, where the individual is not allowed outside of the quarantine facility. Strict quarantine can be as much for the safety of the individual in quarantine as for the protection of the public, guarding against intrusions of aggressive media, political agitators, and even panicked citizens.

To protect and care for the quarantined individual, a quarantine unit should provide not only physical security as above but also adequate access to health care, mental health services, family and social interaction, spiritual services, entertainment, and exercise. Many quarantined individuals may be recently repatriated from working in outbreak, humanitarian disaster, or other stressful settings. These individuals may be suffering from physical exhaustion, sleep deprivation, psychological stress related to their recent environment, jet lag, and anxiety about their potential exposure. In addition, as quarantine periods can last several weeks for some diseases, the facility will need to accommodate these needs for extended periods of time.

Location and Design

Ideally, a quarantine facility is located in a spot with easy access by road and air (to facilitate transportation to and from) with reliable supporting infrastructure, such as power, water, supply chain, and so on, and in proximity to health care resources that can be employed for care during quarantine and in the event that the person becomes symptomatic and must be moved to isolation care. Easy access to a public health reference laboratory is also desirable to facilitate rapid diagnostic testing turnaround. Finally, co-location with a patient isolation/biocontainment unit can expedite transfer to an appropriate level of care in the event that the person does develop disease.

Physical design of a quarantine unit can vary. A quarantine unit should include adequate physical security and access control. If located in hospitals or other busy facilities, more remote wings or even standalone buildings removed from high-traffic areas are optimal. Discrete, negative pressure, or filtered air-handling systems are generally not necessary, nor is special liquid or solid waste handling, as persons who are considered infectious or who have symptoms move from quarantine to isolation. Nevertheless, these additional levels of containment have been added to some quarantine units to enhance public confidence and provide additional layers of controls.

Quarantine space should be outfitted for long-term stays, with rooms designed to provide comfort with hotel-level amenities, including private bathroom and storage space. A homelike feel can significantly ease the stress and anxiety of quarantine. Units should provide phone, internet, and other tools for entertainment and communication with family and friends. Exercise equipment is critical to maintaining physical and mental health during long stays. Room designs should accommodate individuals with disabilities and facilitate providing quarantine to individuals of all ages, including children. Units can provide designated areas in which to receive family, as well as audio and visual capabilities that enable families to communicate with quarantined individuals in circumstances where in-person visitation cannot be arranged. The unit should include laundry and nourishment services.

The unique requirements of quarantine are quite different from isolation. While a patient isolation unit may seem like a ready shortcut for a quarantine unit, we have found that facility design and the level of amenities of an isolation unit provide a poor environment for quarantine. Additionally, if a quarantined person were to become ill and require isolation, the unit would then be unavailable for further quarantine individuals.

Organizational Structure and Coordination

Since quarantine spaces would likely be used on a sporadic rather than a routine basis, yet would need to be activated quickly, they require an organizational and operational structure that is scalable, fast, efficient, and executable. In order to maintain a state of readiness to activate, the quarantine unit must have the following:

1. Well-structured organizational chart with clear and defined levels of authority, roles, and responsibilities.

2. Well-drafted operational plan that includes all necessary standard operating procedures (SOPs).

3. Clearly designed and tested notification plan that can be executed at any time.

Due to the complex and often high-profile nature of transport and care of quarantined individuals, the quarantine unit must maintain close partnership with organizations at the city, county, state, and federal levels, including the city/county health department, state department of health, local fire/police/EMS, political leadership, and others.

Quarantine unit plans should account for a variety of needs related and unrelated to the potential exposure in question. A quarantine unit should have staff available 24/7, preferably on-site, although remote and on-call service could be entertained in some cases. Plans should provide routine outpatient health care services to address chronic medical conditions as well as any acute illness that may be encountered with returning travelers. These plans should include access to laboratory and pharmacy services.

Finally, quarantine unit plans should provide for routine monitoring for symptoms or signs of illness, relevant for the particular disease in question. Monitoring may involve temperature checks, questionnaires, physical assessment, or laboratory testing. Predesignated and exercised protocols can facilitate coordination and smooth operations during a quarantine event.

Conclusion

Most quarantine in the United States is handled at local levels, but the federal government has quarantine authorities as well. In the circumstance of highly dangerous pathogens or other special conditions, dedicated quarantine units may be useful resources. Quarantine units require careful design, plans, training, and implementation to be able to deliver quarantine services in emergencies and to protect the public from spread of disease and provide adequate care for individuals in the charge of the quarantine unit. The National Quarantine Unit at the University of Nebraska Medical Center is a one-of-a-kind asset that stands as an additional tool in the nation's armamentarium and will serve as a national resource for education and training in quarantine operations.

CHAPTER 6

Management of the Person Under Investigation

MICHAEL C. WADMAN
MICHELLE M. SCHWEDHELM

Triage, Travel, and Symptom Screening

A person under investigation (PUI) is defined as an individual with clinical signs and symptoms consistent with the specific disease under consideration, possible exposure history or travel to a designated "hot spot" country within a defined period of time, and a candidate for enhanced precautions and isolation. A PUI may present to a health care facility via the emergency department (ED), clinics, direct admission, emergency medical services (EMS), or various other means. In 2014, as the Ebola outbreak escalated in West Africa, US health care facilities made preparations to identify and appropriately manage patients presenting to their health care facility who may have traveled to West Africa and had symptoms that matched the Centers for Disease Control and Prevention (CDC) case definition for Ebola virus disease (EVD). Since that time, several other highly hazardous communicable disease (HHCD) outbreaks have demonstrated the critical need for health care facilities to develop and implement systems to screen and manage these patients appropriately, while mitigating risks to health care personnel and preventing disruptions in the care of other patients.

Identify, Isolate, Inform

Many hospitals have developed effective strategies to manage prospective PUIs for a variety of HHCDs, and immediate, safe identification of PUIs is the first critical step in the process. "Identify, Isolate, Inform" (3I) is the process model established by CDC for use at front doors of health care facilities. Initial development and implementation of the 3I model focused on presentations of EVD, but this process is easily modified to address other emerging public health threats.

Identification of the PUI

Identification of symptomatic travelers, the initial step in the process, is rapidly implemented in a brief screening process as the patient presents at front desk intake areas. In 2014 most health care facilities initiated this process with a paper screening tool and a map of Africa. One example of this process utilized a paper-based travel and symptom tool in the ED administered by a "greeter" nurse. The greeter nurse, positioned at the front door, was the first contact for any patient seeking care. A travel questionnaire, focusing on the previous 21 days, was aligned with a defined set of at-risk West African countries and presenting symptoms consistent with the CDC case definition for Ebola. Subsequently, analogous screening processes were instituted in other areas of access to the health care facility. ED volume demands resulted in multiple challenges for the paper-based process, however, which led to efforts (with the assistance of information technology experts from the electronic health record [EHR] team) to design and implement an electronic screening solution. The electronic solution design first queried a patient about travel outside the country in the past 21 days, then permitted selection of a specific country. If a country identified was at risk for Ebola, then travel dates were requested and entered. Symptoms (e.g., fever, cough, diarrhea, etc.) described in chief complaint questioning were then entered into the electronic screening tool using point-and-click methodology. If travel history and symptoms matched the CDC Ebola case definition, an automatic alert banner directed the notification of others (e.g., charge nurse, infection prevention personnel) and drove subsequent actions

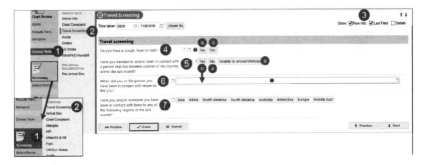

Figure 6.1. 2019 Travel and Symptom Screening Tool (Courtesy of Nebraska Medicine)

(e.g., patient dons mask, caregivers don personal protective equipment [PPE], patient moved to private room, etc.). Travel and symptom screening updates to the EHR have evolved on an ongoing basis since 2014, and screening for other highly hazardous communicable pathogens such as Middle Eastern respiratory syndrome (MERS) coronavirus was added to the tool's capability in 2016. The most recent best practice change includes a combined Ebola and MERS screening via the EHR (see figure 6.1). The first question asked is "Do you have a cough, fever, or rash?" If the patient answers "Yes," a mask is provided to begin the isolation process. This strategy mitigates transmission of numerous communicable diseases in busy waiting rooms (e.g., measles, influenza, special pathogens) as an overall benefit. The screening process then continues with travel questions (using a one-month time frame for simplicity). Hot spot countries are then identified and subsequent alerts provided if symptoms and positive travel screen are identified. The applicable pathogen banner alert message is displayed to encourage the clinician to isolate the patient and then proceed to inform others that the patient may be infected with a special pathogen.

Travel and symptom screening is a single point in the process of triage for special pathogens such as Ebola or MERS coronavirus at health care entry areas. Process and workflow algorithms, to include accountability, action steps, resources, and contact information, are administrative controls to assist the care team in proper isolation, PPE selection, diagnostic testing, and communication (see appendix A at the end of this chapter). Resource examples such as these can be made available at all times via hospital intranet or other electronic system. Administrative controls such as algorithms and checklists are used to provide guidance at all key steps of the Isolation and Inform process.

Isolation, Evaluation, and Management of the PUI

Following identification of the patient as a PUI, isolation of the patient, protection of health care workers, and provision of medical care must all occur in an organized and timely manner. Isolation of the PUI begins with implementation of precautions at the triage area or front desk point of identification. Health care workers attending to the patient when the risk is identified should immediately don appropriate PPE. A procedure mask is placed on the PUI to reduce the likelihood of generating infectious secretions, droplets, or aerosols. Staff should maintain positive control over PUI movement at all times, including having the patient escorted to the isolation area. The isolation area is identified and organized in advance. The space should include 2–3 rooms, if possible, with a private restroom. The patient care room should have negative pressure air flow, and ideally, adjacent rooms would be available for equipment storage and waste sequestration (if designated as category A waste infectious substances, e.g., Ebola). The patient care isolation room should be equipped with a telemedicine link allowing audio and visual communication between the patient and personnel both inside and outside of the patient care room. To assist the clinical team, a pathogen-specific algorithm may be initiated, which guides the step-by-step process to include an infectious disease consult, as well as notification of the health department and public health laboratory for the jurisdiction (appendix A). When direct contact with the patient is required, designated personnel don appropriate PPE as indicated for the infectious agent. A clean zone is established outside of the defined isolation hot zone where a log is kept of personnel who enter the patient's room and where donning of PPE is performed with a donning partner to ensure adherence to the identified protocol.

PUI status must not compromise the appropriate evaluation and management of the patient. The differential diagnosis for PUIs with possible EVD or MERS may include common conditions such as bacterial pneumonia or pyelonephritis, but also exotic infectious diseases such as malaria, meningococcemia, tick-borne rickettsiae, dengue, leptospirosis, and acute schistosomiasis. Many of these diseases may result in significant morbidity and mortality if not diagnosed and treated in a timely manner. A focused physical examination directed by the patient's history and presenting symptoms, followed by a diagnostic workup addressing the appropriate differential diagnosis for each patient, is essential to quality care and mitigates the risk of delayed evaluation and management of a condition unrelated to the PUI status. Monitoring the PUI also requires physical examination data to ensure diagnostic accuracy and to assess the efficacy of any therapeutic interventions. The physical examination performed in PPE is aided by the use of a wireless stethoscope using earbuds inserted prior to donning, as the use of a standard disposable stethoscope adds risk of self-contamination when adjusting or disengaging the earpieces. PUI status remains in effect until final testing for the infectious agent triggering the PUI status is negative. The timing for confirmatory testing varies among infectious agents, and specific recommendations regarding testing regimens are discussed in chapter 17 of this manual. Laboratory testing must follow strict protocols to ensure the safety of the technicians obtaining and running the samples. Laboratory tests include screening for the infectious agent triggering the PUI status and other testing required for patient evaluation and monitoring.

If the PUI requires radiographic evaluation, bedside imaging is preferred. For portable plain radiography, the mobile radiography machine is covered with a surgical drape and the cassette is placed in a plastic sleeve. After the image is obtained, the sleeve is cleaned with bleach, and the cassette is then transferred to the technician for digital transmission of the images from the patient care room. The machine remains in a storage room within the isolation zone for future use or decontamination as dictated by final testing. Bedside testing is also preferred for ultrasound and follows a similar machine draping, with plastic sheath probe cover, and post-imaging storage procedure.

PUIs may occasionally require further diagnostic and therapeutic procedures while awaiting confirmatory testing, and it is essential to consider specific modifications of the most likely procedures in order to ensure patient access to these interventions as well as the safety of personnel performing the procedures. This is especially true for emergency interventions such as airway management and central vascular access, since the risk of exposure is high. A transportation plan should be developed to move PUIs from isolation to a diagnostic location and procedures for cleaning the diagnostic space as appropriate to the pathogen should be defined.

Airway interventions, such as bag-valve-mask ventilation and tracheal intubation, increase the risk of dermal and respiratory exposure to aerosolized saliva and blood. For those requiring intubation, in order to reduce the potential for aerosolized fluid, rapid sequence induction with full neuromuscular blockade is recommended to eliminate the formation of aerosols from coughing or emesis. Laryngoscopy using video technologies is favored over direct techniques so that the distance from patient airway to provider is maximized to reduce exposure risk. While defined PPE provides full coverage necessary to prevent aerosols from settling on exposed skin of the neck or face, powered air-purifying respirators are used during all airway interventions to prevent the inhalation of fine aerosols. Additional guidance on the performance of medical procedures on patients with HHCDs is provided in chapter 9.

Exercises are essential to hardwire processes that are high-risk and low-probability occurrences. Opportunities to manage PUIs are typically infrequent, but represent opportunities to revise and improve tools, resources, and care practices. The National Ebola Training and Education Center (NETEC) has a robust suite of exercise templates at www.netec.org that are helpful in the identification, assessment, treatment, transportation, and/or transfer of special pathogen patients. These templates are fully customizable, approved by the Assistant Secretary of Preparedness & Response (ASPR) and the CDC, and based on the Homeland Security Exercise and Evaluation Program (HSEEP) model.

Appropriate management of the PUI is a challenge to health care facilities and caregivers. However, a robust travel and symptom screening strategy, the availability of predefined workflow algorithms, team training to include proper use of PPE, and an occasional mystery patient exercise can go a long way in making this challenge a safe and manageable situation.

Appendix A

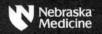

LOCATION	ROLE	PROCESS STEP	NOTES

ED Front Desk — Greeter/Triage Nurse

1 PATIENT HISTORY GATHERED
Ask: Do you have a fever, cough or rash?
*one symptom considered positive

YES — Provide Patient Mask and Continue with Travel Questions

NO — Continue with Travel Questions

MERS Co-V Outbreak Areas
www.cdc.gov/coronavirus/mers/

Case Definition: Compatible MERS Co-V Symptoms = fever >100.4F/38C, cough, SOB OR pneumonia/ARDS (based on clinical or radiological evidence
www.cdc.gov/coronavirus/mers/case-def.html

Greeter/Triage Nurse

2 TRAVEL QUESTION
Have you traveled to and/or been in contact with a person that has traveled outside of the country within the last month?

NO STOP

YES

! CLOSE CONTACT
is defined as (a) being within approximately 6 feet or within the room or care area for a prolonged period of time while not wearing recommended PPE or (b) having direct contact with infectious secretions (e.g., being coughed on) while not wearing PPE.

Greeter/Triage Nurse

3 If yes, to what country? If patient traveled to hot spot, notify lead nurse

NO STOP

If patient arrives with family member(s):

Greeter/Triage Nurse

4 FAMILY HISTORY GATHERED
Does family member have **ANY** of the MERS Co-V symptoms listed above?

NO

YES

Escort family to family conference room

If any family member is symptomatic, room E6 will be used as a second "patient room" for that individual

Decisions on where to house asymptomatic family/friends will be left to the discretion of the triage nurse and be based on the needs of the patient.

Greeter/Triage Nurse

5 Provide family members procedure masks and gloves and instructs on how to apply.

LOCATION	ROLE	PROCESS STEP	NOTES
	Greeter/Triage Nurse	**6** Ask ED front desk staff to call lead nurse to (1) report positive history/symptoms and (2) check on availability of rooms E6 through E8.	
	Lead Nurse	Rooms E6 through E8 available? ···· **NO** ········ **YES**	Clear and disinfect rooms
	Greeter/Triage Nurse	**7** Escort patient(s) to room E7. Instruct patient to (1) remain in room, (2) keep door closed and (3) that a nurse will be with them as soon as she/he has a proper PPE.	
	Lead Nurse	**8** Establish who will serve in each of the following roles: (1) primary nurse, (2) task.	
Rooms E6-8	Lead Nurse	**9** (1) Tape "Do Not Enter" sign to patient room, (2) Tape "Room Entry Log" to patient room and (3) Tape "Soiled Utility" sign to appropriate room.	**See ED 24-hour sheet for on-call manager contact information**
	Lead Nurse / ED Manager On Call	**10** Notify ED manager on call of possible MERS Co-V patient. Notify Infection Control (IC) liaison (XXX.XXX.XXXX) of possible MERS Co-V patient. Notify Security of need for personnel to control entry to designated rooms.	**!** **Security to monitor entry to isolation area round the clock** **!** MERS CO-V Lab Go kits are located in Triage C.
Isolation Room	Primary Nurse / Primary Nurse / Task Nurse / Lead Nurse	**11** *Primary nurse* – Picks up MERS Co-V lab kit and gather MERS Co-V PPE. *Task nurse* – Don level PPE for MERS Co-V. *Lead nurse* – Observe donning process.	Gather MERS CO-V PPE: Yellow isolation gown Face shield/goggles 2 pair gloves–(nitrile gloves as base glove; regular patient care gloves over the nitrile) N-95 respirator for general care **PAPR when performing aerosol generating procedures**

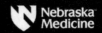

LOCATION	ROLE	PROCESS STEP	NOTES
Isolation Room	Primary Nurse	**12** Gather full set of vitals and any additional pertinent information.	Logs are located in the MERS book. All people entering room must sign in on "Room Entry Log" before each entry into the isolation room.
	ER Attending Task Nurse	**13** Don MERS Co-V PPE. Observe donning process.	Routine blood labs may be drawn at any point during encounter, but must be processed for transport per MERS Co-V lab protocol.
Isolation Room	ER Attending	**14** Examine/assess patient.	

14 Examine/assess patient.

In the 14 days before symptom onset did the patient:
1. Travel to or from the Arabian Peninsula/ neighboring countries? If yes, which countries?
2. Exact date of travel **to** stated area. Exact date of travel **from** stated area.
3. Visit or work in a health care facility in the Arabian Peninsula/neighboring country? If yes, which countries? **Is the patient a health care worker?**
4. Have close contact with an ill traveler from the Arabian Peninsula/neighboring country? If yes, which countries?
5. **Is the patient a member of a severe respiratory illness cluster of unknown etiology?**
6. Have close contact with a **known** MERS case? **Had close contact with a camel?**

Table 1

CLINICAL FEATURES		EPIDEMIOLOGIC RISK
1) Severe illness Fever *and* pneumonia or acute respiratory distress syndrome (based on clinical or radiological evidence)	AND	A history of travel from countries in or near the Arabian Peninsula within 14 days before symptom onset, or close contact with a symptomatic traveler who developed fever and acute respiratory illness (not necessarily pneumonia) within 14 days after traveling from countries in or near the Arabian Peninsula. *– or –* A member of a cluster of patients with severe acute respiratory illness (e.g., fever and pneumonia requiring hospitalization) of unknown etiology in which MERS-CoV is being evaluated, in consultation with state and local health departments in the U.S.
2) Milder illness Fever *or* symptoms of respiratory illness (not necessarily pneumonia; e.g., cough, shortness of breath)	AND	Close contact with a confirmed MERS case while the case was ill. *– or –* A history of being in a health care facility (as a patient, worker, or visitor) within 14 days before symptom onset in a country or territory in or near the Arabian Peninsula in which recent health care-associated cases of MERS have been identified.
3) Milder illness Fever *or* symptoms of respiratory illness (not necessarily pneumonia; e.g., cough, shortness of breath	AND	History of travel to a country or territory in or near the Arabian Peninsula.

Case Definition: Compatible MERS Co-V symptoms = fever >100.4F/38C, cough, SOB OR pneumonia/ARDS (based on clinical or radiological evidence *www.cdc.gov/coronavirus/ mers/case-def.html*

LOCATION	ROLE	PROCESS STEP	NOTES

15 Patient meets clinical criteria 1 or 2 from table 1 (page 3).

YES NO

!

If patient meets clinical criteria 3 from table 1, order Respiratory Pathogen Panel (RPP). If RPP positive, treatment per ED attending. If RPP is negative, proceed to step 16.

ER Attending

16 Call ID attending MD for academic general ID service on call for consult **(ID MD)**

ID MD

17a Notifies Nebraska Biocontainment Unit (NBU) medical director if either clinical criteria 1 or 2 is met.

17b Arrange for lab testing by Nebraska Public Health Lab (NPHL).

Isolation Room

Primary Nurse

18 Collect specimen/draw blood to send to NPHL per MERS Co-V protocol. NPHL staff will pick up specimen(s).

ID MD

Enter orders for lab in OneChart: "Special Procedure: Other."

MERS Co-V specimens for NPHL analysis must be processed per *MERS Co-V lab draw protocol*

Lab

19 Call ED medical director, ID medical director and NBU medical director with results.

20 MERS Co-V PCR test presumptive positive?

YES NO

ED lead phone XXX.XXX.XXXX

If specimen is negative, NPHL will reflex appropriate specimen to Core lab for RPP if not already performed. Patient is admitted or discharged dependent on clinical picture.

LOCATION	ROLE	PROCESS STEP	NOTES
	ID MD	**21** Notify NBU medical director of presumptive positive result.	
	ED Lead	**22** Notify ED manager and IC on call laision at XXX.XXX.XXXX of presumptive positive result.	
	ED Attending	**23** If PUI refuses care: ID medical director to call state/county public health director to obtain isolation.	Local Health Department Days: XXX.XXX.XXXX After 4:30 p.m.: XXX.XXX.XXXX
	ED Manager On Call	**24** Notify Public Information Officer (PIO) and Nebraska Medicine Incident Commander on call.	
		25 Activate NBU for transport to NBU.	

CHAPTER 7

Isolation in the Conventional Hospital Setting

L. KATE TYNER
ANGELA L. HEWLETT

Introduction

Isolation is a fundamental principle of routine infection control practice that is utilized with the intent of preventing the spread of infection in health care settings. Isolation of patients with confirmed or suspected infectious diseases provides a method to reduce or prevent exposure to infectious agents among patients, health care workers, and others in the health care environment. Isolation procedures are separated into standard precautions, which apply to all patients, and transmission-based precautions, which apply to patients infected or colonized with certain pathogens. Although the general principles of standard precautions should be applied to patients in all settings, transmission-based isolation precautions may vary significantly among facilities. Thus, isolation practices may be dependent on the type of health care setting (acute-care hospital, long-term care facility, dialysis center, etc.), environmental controls (private vs. shared rooms, negative pressure rooms), organizational characteristics (staffing, availability of personal protective equipment [PPE]), local epidemiology and resistance patterns, and other issues. Transmission-based isolation precautions

Table 7.1 Standard Precautions. Adapted from CDC Guideline for Isolation Precautions: Preventing Transmission of Infectious Agents in Health Care Settings (2007).

Perform hand hygiene
Use of personal protective equipment (PPE) whenever there is an expectation of possible exposure to infectious material
Utilize principles of respiratory hygiene and cough etiquette
Place patients who pose a transmission risk to others in a single room if available
Develop procedures for environmental cleaning, as well as the cleaning and disinfection of patient care equipment, instruments, and devices between patient use
Handle textiles and laundry carefully to prevent the transfer of microorganisms
Follow safe injection practices and handle needles and sharp devices carefully

may be instituted in an empirical fashion when there is concern for infection or colonization with a specific pathogen, or may be syndromic, based on the clinical presentation of the patient. This chapter will discuss various routine isolation practices and their applicability in the health care setting.

Standard Precautions

Standard precautions are infection control principles that are applied to all patients in all health care settings in order to decrease the risk of transmission of infectious diseases. Standard precautions are detailed in table 7.1.

Transmission-based Precautions

Transmission-based precautions include contact precautions, droplet precautions, and airborne precautions. These are utilized for patients with known or suspected communicable diseases in order to decrease the risk of transmission to health care workers and other patients.

Contact Precautions

The indications for the use of contact precautions are highly variable among facilities. Contact precautions are generally used for patients who are infected or colonized with multidrug-resistant organisms (MDROs) spread by direct contact or contact with fomites, the most problematic of which include vancomycin-resistant enterococci (VRE), methicillin-resistant *Staphylococcus aureus* (MRSA), and multidrug-resistant *Enterobacteriaceae* (MDR-E), such as extended spectrum beta-lactamase producing organisms and carbapenem-resistant *Enterobacteriaceae*. Other indications may include gastroenteritis (e.g., norovirus, *Clostridioides difficile*), draining wounds, parainfluenza, lice, respiratory syncytial virus (RSV), scabies, and *Burkholderia cepacia* in patients with cystic fibrosis.

PATIENT PLACEMENT

A single patient space or room is preferred to decrease the risk of transmission to other patients. If a single patient space is not available, cohorting patients known to have the same infection or colonizing agent can be considered, based on conditions that are associated with transmission such as incontinence or drainage that cannot be contained.

PERSONAL PROTECTIVE EQUIPMENT

Gowns and gloves should be worn when contact with the patient and the patient's environment is expected, and removed before leaving the patient space.

LIMITING PATIENT TRANSPORT

Movement of the patient outside of the room should be limited to medical necessity. When movement is necessary, the infected or colonized part of the patient should be covered with a clean gown and cover sheet. Contaminated PPE should be removed and disposed of, and hand hygiene performed prior to transport. Clean PPE should be donned at the transport location when providing care for the patient. Administrative controls, such as alerts in the electronic medical record and signage, should be used to assist with communication about the need for transmission-based precautions.

If equipment cannot be dedicated, then it should be cleaned and disinfected before being used on another patient. Disposable patient care equipment should also be considered.

The rooms of patients on contact precautions should be cleaned and disinfected at least daily, with a focus on surfaces that are touched frequently by the patient and health care workers. Ensure that disinfectants are effective against the organism of concern by ensuring that the label includes an organism inactivation claim. Ensure that disinfectant manufacturers' instructions for use are followed, especially as they apply to contact time and preparation. Environmental service workers should use gowns and gloves for room cleaning and disinfection.

Droplet Precautions

GENERAL INDICATIONS FOR USE

Common indications include but are not limited to *Bordetella pertussis*, influenza virus, adenovirus, rhinovirus, *Neisseria meningitidis*, and certain group A streptococcal infections.

PATIENT PLACEMENT

A single patient space or room is preferred to decrease the risk of transmission to other patients. If a single patient space is not available, cohorting patients known to have the same infection or colonizing agent can be considered based on conditions that are associated with transmission such as respiratory secretions that are excessive or cannot be contained. Patients should be separated by at least 6 feet with privacy curtains drawn. Immunosuppressed patients should not be cohorted with patients on droplet precautions.

Don a surgical mask before entering the patient's room or space.

LIMIT PATIENT TRANSPORT

Movement of the patient outside of the room should be limited to medical necessity. When movement is necessary, instruct the patient to wear a surgical mask and adhere to respiratory hygiene and principles of cough etiquette. Administrative controls, such as alerts in the electronic medical record and signage, should be used to assist with communication about the need for transmission-based precautions.

SOURCE CONTROL

Until appropriate patient placement and isolation is established, the patient should wear a surgical mask if medically tolerated.

Airborne Precautions

GENERAL INDICATIONS FOR USE

Common indications for airborne isolation include patients with suspected or confirmed tuberculosis, measles, chicken pox, or disseminated herpes zoster.

PATIENT PLACEMENT

Airborne infection isolation rooms (AIIRs) should be equipped with special air handling and ventilation capacity that meet the American Institute of Architects/Facility Guidelines Institute (AIA/FGI) standards for AIIRs (i.e., monitored negative pressure relative to the surrounding area, 12 air exchanges per hour for new construction and renovation and 6 air exchanges per hour for existing facilities, air exhausted directly to the outside or recirculated through HEPA filtration before return). If an appropriately engineered room is not available, the patient should be instructed to don a surgical mask and placed in a private room with the door closed until the patient is transferred to a facility with an appropriate room or returned home (if condition allows and with public health notification).

Health care workers should wear a fit-tested National Institute for Occupational Safety and Health (NIOSH)–approved N95 (or higher-level) respirator when caring for patients in airborne isolation.

LIMIT PATIENT TRANSPORT

Movement of the patient outside of the room should be limited to medical necessity. When movement out of the airborne infection isolation room is necessary, a surgical mask should be placed on the patient and the patient instructed to adhere to respiratory hygiene and principles of cough etiquette. Administrative controls, such as alerts in the electronic medical record and signage, should be used to assist with communication about the need for transmission-based precautions. If the patient is wearing a mask and infectious skin lesions are covered, then the health care workers do not need to wear a mask during transport.

SOURCE CONTROL

Until appropriate patient placement and isolation is established, the patient should wear a surgical mask if medically tolerated.

Conclusion

Isolation, including both standard and transmission-based precautions, is an important part of routine infection control practice in health care settings. Although there is evidence to support the utilization of isolation precautions to reduce the risk of disease transmission, it is important to note that some degree of controversy exists over which pathogens necessitate isolation. For instance, some facilities screen for and implement contact isolation for patients colonized with MRSA, while others use standard precautions for these patients. Although a full discussion of the controversies in isolation practice is beyond the scope of this chapter, decisions regarding the need for isolation of patients should be made after consideration of the available scientific evidence, environmental and facility issues, and local epidemiologic data. It is important to note that isolation of patients with known or suspected infectious diseases is only one component of a comprehensive infection control program, and should always be utilized in conjunction with other evidence-based measures such as hand hygiene and environmental cleaning in order to prevent the spread of infection in the health care environment.

CHAPTER 8

High-Level Containment Care Unit Operations

AURORA B. LE
JOHN J. LOWE
SCOTT J. PATLOVICH
ROBERT EMERY
ELIZABETH L. BEAM
JAMES V. LAWLER
AMANDA STRAIN
ANGELA M. VASA
MICHELLE M. SCHWEDHELM
SHAWN G. GIBBS

High-level containment care (HLCC) refers to the management of patients with highly hazardous communicable diseases (HHCDs) performed in specialized clinical biocontainment units that possess a variety of controls to prevent transmission of infection while facilitating effective patient care. However, the presence of a purpose-built patient care unit does not guarantee safe and effective care of HHCDs, nor is it an indispensable component of such care. The foundation of HLCC is a well-trained team of providers adhering to core principles of operation, such as the hierarchy of controls. This chapter explores the fundamentals of HLCC operations and the application of hierarchy for the care of HHCD patients, along with other key concepts.

Infection control and biocontainment practices in HLCC units are implemented by interdisciplinary teams with competency in patient care, biosafety, infection control, and the utilization of personal protective equipment (PPE). These practices emphasize pathogen containment in order to reduce and limit health care worker (HCW) exposures while enabling the provision of advanced critical care. HCWs require time and training to develop competencies in their organization's standard operating procedures (SOPs) and transmission-based infection control practice within the biocontainment unit environment. With education and training comes deeper knowledge of the nuances of HHCD care, mastery of the principles of HLCC, and confidence in the appropriate execution of protocols.

The safe care for patients with HHCDs utilizes a combination of effective biosafety and infection control practices that extends well beyond negative pressure rooms and PPE. Although HLCC units incorporate many of the engineering designs and industrial hygiene standards developed for laboratory biosafety (most closely reflecting laboratory biosafety level 3), they must also provide an environment conducive to patient care and recovery. Human factors associated with HCW comfort, safety, and effectiveness also weigh heavily in the development of protocols and selection of PPE and other equipment. The provision of safe HLCC care requires extensive prior planning, development, and implementation of administrative policies, work practices, and environmental controls.

Key Concepts: Zones of Risk and Movement within the Biocontainment Unit

Actions within HLCC settings are predicated on the concept of zones of risk. To create standard frames of reference, risk of pathogen contamination is geographically defined, and protocols and activities are dictated by the zone in which they reside. Spaces in the HLCC unit where confirmed/infected patients reside (e.g., isolation rooms) constitute the area of highest risk. Administrative areas, completely separated from isolation rooms by physical and engineering barriers, are areas of negligible risk. These different areas are often described by a variety of naming systems, such as "dirty" and "clean," "hot" and "cold," or "red" and "green."

Naming schemes can inject gradations of risk as well, such as "warm" or "yellow."

Facility design and operation should promote unidirectional movement of personnel, equipment, and supplies into and out of the facility whenever possible, ideally moving from zones of lower to higher risk and then egressing through a process of doffing and decontamination. On entry to the HLCC unit, staff move into an anteroom that allows them to don the appropriate PPE ensemble for the activities to be performed. All personal items, jewelry, watches, and other nonessential items are left in the anteroom or outside the facility altogether. Entry into the high-level containment patient care area occurs after verification of correct donning of all PPE. Movement within the unit should proceed from zones of lowest to highest risk, or warm to hot. Personnel should avoid backtracking to zones of lower risk, and protocols and procedures should reflect this concept.

Egress from the high-risk area and associated doffing of PPE presents one of the most significant opportunities for self-contamination of HCWs. Based on the lessons learned from Dallas in 2014, where two health care workers contracted Ebola virus disease (EVD) during patient care, it is imperative that all personnel are trained and drill frequently on the proper doffing process to prevent cross contamination. Suggested procedures for donning and doffing are detailed later in this chapter. The use of a trained observer is also recommended by the Centers for Disease Control and Prevention (CDC) for this process to assist personnel leaving the biocontainment facility.

The Hierarchy of Controls

The industrial hygiene concept of the hierarchy of controls (HoC) is instrumental in the management of individuals with a suspected or confirmed HHCD (see figure 8.1). The concept of HoC is used throughout industry to minimize occupational exposures to hazards, and its implementation in HLCC creates the foundation of effective biocontainment. Regardless of whether the pathogen of concern is transmitted via the airborne, droplet, or contact route, each level of the hierarchy—*elimination, substitution, engineering controls, administrative controls,* and *PPE*—

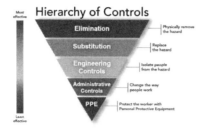

Hierarchy of Controls

Elimination — Physically remove the hazard

Substitution — Replace the hazard

Engineering Controls — Isolate people from the hazard

Administrative Controls — Change the way people work

PPE — Protect the worker with Personal Protective Equipment

Most effective

Least effective

Figure 8.1. The Hierarchy of Controls (Figure by NIOSH)

must be considered with respect to its role in minimizing hazard and optimizing care. One should note that the HoC is indeed a hierarchy, proceeding in order of importance and effectiveness. Elimination of the hazard is always preferred as the most effective intervention, with substitution being the next most effective, although these options obviously are not always possible with respect to pathogens in an HLCC unit. At the bottom of the HoC, PPE is considered the least effective modality. It is a last line of defense, the effectiveness of which depends on proper usage and maintenance, selection of equipment, fit, donning and doffing technique, and operation. Finally, the HoC applies to all hazards in the HLCC environment—such as techniques for pathogen decontamination—and should shape decisions for all protocols and activities occurring within the biocontainment unit.

ELIMINATION

Essentially, HLCC units functionally achieve elimination of HHCD pathogens for hospitals and health systems by removing them from the standard health care environment. As noted, however, this means that complete pathogen elimination is not possible within HLCC. Nevertheless, opportunities exist to eliminate unnecessary points of exposure. Elimination efforts also should address hazards other than the HHCD pathogen.

Stepwise processes within HLCC often present opportunities to eliminate pathogen hazards upstream. For example, infectious patient specimens can be inactivated and nucleic acids extracted at the bedside or within the HLCC unit prior to transportation to a clinical laboratory. During the 2014–16 West Africa Ebola outbreak, HLCC units used a variety of procedures to inactivate Ebola virus in clinical specimens. Establishing a satellite clinical laboratory inside the unit, including a biosafety cabinet, centrifuge, and other necessary equipment can eliminate the need to transport some specimens outside of the unit altogether.

Selection of disinfectants and other chemicals present additional opportunity for hazard elimination within HLCC units. For instance, while the US Environmental Protection Agency (EPA) approves both quaternary ammonium and sodium hypochlorite (bleach) disinfectants against various HHCD pathogens, improper use of these agents in combination can generate toxic chloramine gas. Eliminating one of these classes of agents from standard procedures can remove the potential for chloramine exposure within HLCC.

SUBSTITUTION

Substitution is the second-most effective means to control hazards and entails replacing a hazard with a comparable process with reduced risk. As with elimination, pathogen substitution is not applicable for HLCC, but substitution is a key method of control related to other hazards in the HLCC unit.

For example, substitution of alternative decontamination procedures, such as vaporized hydrogen peroxide or ultraviolet germicidal irradiation (UVGI), can prevent exposure to more hazardous compounds (e.g., formaldehyde). Instead of chemical dunk tanks or sprayers, such as sodium hypochlorite, substitution of sodium hypochlorite wipes for decontamination of medical equipment could eliminate slip hazards. Physical hazards are often overlooked in HLCC environments, but they are major sources of potential direct injury or breach of PPE. Due to the sensory, movement, and dexterity restrictions associated with PPE, staff within the unit are more vulnerable to such hazards. Liquid disinfectants can create significant slip hazards when applied to flooring, and this hazard can be moderated by substitution of lower volume/more rapidly drying decontamination methods (wipes) or footwear and floor surfaces with higher coefficients of friction. Moreover, sharp edges and pinch points can lead to physical trauma as well as PPE breach and pathogen exposure, and they present important opportunities for hazard substitution. HLCC unit design should consider alternatives to shelves and other wall decor that can serve as bump or cut hazards. Furniture and equipment should be minimized and selected so as to avoid sharp edges that are likely to catch on PPE. Furniture or building materials made of porous materials (e.g., fabric) should be substituted for nonporous materials to prevent harboring of pathogens.

When drafting supply lists for use in a HLCC unit, teams should look at medical supply options that have the highest safety margin and lowest likelihood of being out of stock during surge periods. Retracting needle systems for syringes and IV catheters can reduce the risk of needle sticks. Needle-less systems of IV infusion kits might reduce risk even further. HLCC protocols should replace any glassware with nonbreakable plastics. Glass ampules, common items in emergency medication kits such as code carts, are particularly hazardous and should be avoided.

ENGINEERING CONTROLS

Engineering controls are design or function features of the physical facility that reduce the odds of HCW exposure to pathogens in the HLCC unit. These features include high-flow negative pressure heating, ventilation, and air-conditioning (HVAC) systems, nonporous finishes on surfaces, physical separation of areas of high risk from low, and others.

Current recommendations for HLCC HVAC systems include a separate air system from the rest of the hospital with a minimum of 12 air exchanges per hour and high-efficiency particle air (HEPA)–filtered exhaust. Exhaust should vent a minimum of 25 feet from any building openings, and dual fans provide redundancy in case of malfunction. Isolation rooms should be negatively pressured at no less than 0.01 inches water gauge (wg) and preferably to 0.03 inches wg compared to noncontainment rooms. HLCC units should have pressure gauges to monitor the pressure continuously in each room, and digital gauges can allow for alarm function and remote monitoring.

Many HLCC units employ a variety of other engineering controls. Floor plans can provide for unidirectional movement of HCWs through the facility from areas of least to greatest contamination, reducing risk of cross contamination. Finish materials with antimicrobial properties can also reduce fomite contamination risk. If UVGI is deployed as part of the decontamination process, UV-reflective paint can be utilized within the HLCC setting to maximize the effect of UVGI. Walls, flooring, and ceiling materials can be engineered and sealed to prevent air and fluids (and pathogens) from exiting the HLCC unit while withstanding surface decontamination with chemical disinfectants. Windows should be sealed to prevent aerosol escape. Built-in, pass-through autoclaves can facilitate safe and efficient disposal of solid waste on-site. The liquid waste system can be designed to allow for storage and disinfection prior to discharge to the wastewater stream.

Details of design and engineering features of HLCC units are well beyond the scope of this text, which is not intended to be an exhaustive reference. Readers who are interested in discussion in more depth should consult some of the published overviews of HLCC unit design (see references), which can serve as a useful starting point for further research.

ADMINISTRATIVE CONTROLS

When engineering controls cannot provide complete protection from exposure, administrative controls such as staffing protocols, SOPs, and training can be used to reduce risk. HLCC operation requires robust administrative support to manage personnel rosters, unit access, training requirements and currencies, equipment maintenance, supply inventory, and curation of SOPs. The combination of these administrative functions should be used to create a *culture of safety* within the organization, a culture that should infuse every training and operation activity.

Standard Operating Procedures. SOPs are key elements in the administrative controls used in a biocontainment unit. The development, practice, and refinement of these protocols form the foundation of the training and exercise program. HLCC team members who participate in training should be encouraged to contribute to the development of the SOPs. Improvement modifications identified during training and exercises should be documented and integrated using a standardized approach. The ability to integrate team members' feedback in an agile fashion will facilitate a deeper understanding of the SOPs and foster a culture of safety and engagement in which staff feel empowered to participate in all aspects of the unit operations.

Telemedicine. The incorporation of telemedicine into HLCC operations is an administrative control that can expand patient access to specialty care and support services while limiting transmission opportunities to other hospital staff and bystanders. Telemedicine, or alternative web-based communication solutions, can be used to complete patient interviews, conduct intermittent assessments, access spiritual support, allow family communications, and provide ancillary services such as physical therapy, occupational therapy, dietetics, and child life. Telemedicine has been used to allow specialty consultation services (e.g., dermatology) to access the patient without having to enter the isolation room. While high-fidelity secure video systems may offer optimal telemedicine capability (particularly for transmission of images or video for diagnostic purposes), secure internet-based video communication platforms using dedicated tablets can provide a more affordable and easier alternative.

Access Control. The HLCC unit should be clearly demarcated and isolated from the rest of the building. A combination of engineering and administrative controls can be used to limit access to high-risk areas and thus reduce chances of accidental exposure of HCWs or bystanders. Entry into the biocontainment unit should be through locked doors, and access should be monitored and limited to only essential, trained, and authorized personnel. Entry controls such as badge-activated access locks and/or biometrics verification with computer-monitored security systems and security officers at the entrance points are typically in place to provide gatekeeping. Signs should be posted to inform nonauthorized personnel of entry restrictions and should include contact information for individuals responsible for and knowledgeable about the facility in case of emergency. Direct access from the exterior of the building is ideal for delivering patients, so that access to the HLCC area does not require comingling with other building operations. If a dual-door system is utilized for entry into the HLCC unit, doors should be interlocked so that the second door will not open until the first is completely closed.

PERSONAL PROTECTIVE EQUIPMENT

With engineering and administrative controls in place, PPE provides a final layer of safety by imposing a barrier between the infectious microorganisms and the human operator. While attention frequently gravitates toward PPE in HLCC operations, experienced staff understand that it represents the last resort of protection. The effectiveness of PPE depends on the selection of appropriate PPE posture and equipment, and it most directly relies on adequate training and proficiency of staff in its use. Generally speaking, a variety of PPE ensembles can be successful in any given situation; however, any poor infection-control behaviors among staff will inevitably result in failure, with potential risks to the individual or others.

Biocontainment units have access to a wide variety of manufacturers and models of PPE approved by appropriate governmental agencies (Food and Drug Administration, National Institute for Occupational Safety and Health, etc.) and manufactured and tested to the proper standards.

In selecting specific PPE products for use in HLCC, leaders should consider the unique needs of their biocontainment unit and a variety of internal and external factors, including:

- Level of protection required for the transmission risk
- Barrier properties of the materials and protection of interfaces
- Durability, fit, and comfort of the equipment
- Ease of use
- Cost and availability

In safety, cost is generally omitted from consideration during PPE selection. However, given the uniqueness of the environment, as well as the high throughput of PPE usage during HLCC care, cost and availability should be a factor.

The US Occupational Safety and Health Administration (OSHA) promulgates standards on blood-borne pathogens, PPE, and respiratory protection (29 CFR 1910.1030; 29 CFR 1910.132; 29 CFR 1910.134) with which employers must comply when preparing employees to care for patients with HHCDs. Leadership should be familiar with these standards and understand the types of PPE available, the training required for reliable protection, and the written procedures necessary. Prior to selecting PPE, HLCC unit leadership should conduct a thorough risk assessment to identify environmental risks to personal safety and health. This assessment should guide selection of individual pieces of equipment that make up the full PPE ensemble. An OSHA PPE selection matrix is provided in figure 8.2.

Selecting Appropriate PPE. Depending on the type and level of pro-

	✔	Use at a minimum
	◆	Use when high(er)-risk exposure(s) is present

	Providing medical and supportive care					
Typical precautions/PPE, if any, for normal work tasks	to individuals with no signs, symptoms, or risk factors for Ebola	to individuals with risk factors for Ebola, but with no signs or symptoms	during initial evaluation of individuals with suspected Ebola (including those with some signs or symptoms), but without obvious bleeding, vomiting, or diarrhea	during initial evaluation of individuals with suspected Ebola who have bleeding, vomiting, or diarrhea, or when these symptoms are likely to develop; or during hospitalization of individuals with suspected or confirmed Ebola	to individuals with suspected or confirmed Ebola, which involves performing aerosol-generating procedures (AGPs)	while transporting sick individuals with risk factors for Ebola or who are suspected or confirmed to have Ebola
	Standard precautions	Standard precautions	Standard precautions	Standard precautions	Standard precautions	Standard precautions
Dedicated clothing (uniform/scrubs, shoes)		◆	✔	✔	✔	✔
Gloves, Single (nitrile)		◆				
Gloves, Double (nitrile)			✔	✔	✔	✔
Gloves, Double (nitrile + heavy duty)						
Face mask (e.g., surgical mask)			✔			
Face and eye protection (e.g., shield/goggles)			✔	✔	✔	✔
Head/neck cover (e.g., surgical hood)[6]				✔ Impermeable	✔ Impermeable	✔ Impermeable
Fluid-resistant or impermeable gown[6]			✔ Fluid-resistant garment should fully cover skin	✔ Appropriate garment should fully cover skin	✔ Impermeable garment should fully cover skin	✔ Impermeable garment should fully cover skin
Fluid-resistant or impermeable coveralls[6]						
Fluid-resistant or impermeable apron[6]			◆ Fluid-resistant	✔ Impermeable	✔ Impermeable	✔ Impermeable
Shoe/boot covers high enough to cover lower leg[6]				✔ Impermeable	✔ Impermeable	✔ Impermeable
Disposable N95 respirator[7]			◆			
Elastomeric respirator + appropriate cartridge[7]			◆	✔	✔	✔
Powered Air-Purifying Respirator (PAPR)[7]			◆			
Full-body, air-supplied positive pressure suit						
Example of workers who may require this level of PPE	Healthcare workers, including physicians, nurses, and others; aid workers; airline and other transportation workers				Healthcare workers, including physicians, nurses, and others	Air medical transport workers, EMS workers

Figure 8.2. OSHA PPE Selection Matrix for Ebola (Figure by OSHA)

tection required, PPE ensembles can include a myriad of equipment options. Because most pathogens require mucus membrane deposit or nonintact skin contact for transmission, equipment to protect the face (especially the mucus membranes) and hands should receive the most attention. Supply orders should account for a variety of sizes. Equipment that does not fit properly creates exposure risks due to physical injuries or unintentional exposure (e.g., tripping on a gown that is too long, tearing a too-tight coverall while squatting, loose-fitting face shield sliding down the face), and ill-fitting equipment is more likely to breach.

Goggles, face shields, respirators, masks, and hoods can be used separately or in combination with other pieces of equipment to protect the face, head, and neck from exposure to pathogens. Eye protection should protect from droplets and splashes at all angles, meaning that common safety glasses are generally inadequate. Although standard surgical masks provide adequate mucous membrane protection for droplet/contact precautions, long-term wear can compromise comfort, particularly if the mask is exposed to sweat or other liquids. Noncollapsible surgical mask products may provide a more comfortable alternative.

Several options exist for respiratory protection in HLCC. Although surgical masks do not protect against airborne or aerosolized particles, placing a surgical mask on an infectious patient, if they can tolerate it, has been shown to reduce the aerosolization of infectious particles into the environment, which protects the HCW. Filtering facepiece respirators (e.g., N95, P100) are disposable respirators that cover the nose and mouth with an air-purifying filter that is tightly fitted and sealed to the face. Half-facepiece and full-facepiece elastomeric respirators (figures 8.3 and 8.4) are reusable respirators with disposable parts. The masks can be cleaned and decontaminated, but the cartridges or canisters used for filtration eventually require replacement. The half- and full-facepiece elastomeric respirators are tightly fitted to the face and sealed around the nose and mouth. Full-facepiece elastomeric respirators have a larger face coverage area and provide eye protection the half-facepiece does not offer, along with a higher assigned protection factor (APF). The filtering facepiece respirator and the half- and full-facepiece elastomeric respirators require fit testing before they are used. Fit testing checks the respirator's seal to the face of the individual being tested, based on the

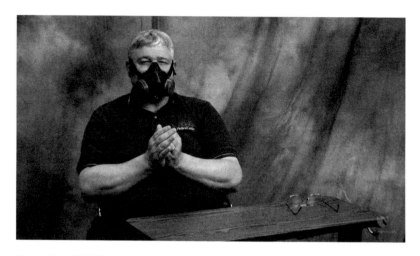

Figure 8.3. Half-Facepiece Respirator (Courtesy of Nebraska Medicine)

respirator model selected, and the stability of the respirator while the individual is moving and talking; workers must only wear respirators for which they have been properly fit tested.

Powered air-purifying respirators (PAPRs) are loose-fitting respirators that use a battery-powered blower to circulate filtered air through the facepiece. PAPRs can be used with a hood or helmet for varying degrees of face, head, and neck protection. The cartridges or canisters attached to the PAPR are disposable but usually last for multiple uses. Batteries for the PAPR blower can be single-use or rechargeable. Loose-fitting PAPRs do not require fit testing and can be used effectively with facial hair, as opposed to most fitted respirators. PAPRs must be assembled and tested to identify safety risks with each use. Respirator use requires attention to many critical aspects, and all HCW and staff wearing them must be part of the organization's respiratory protection and occupational health programs. These programs manage proper fit testing for nonpowered respirators, suitability assessments such as pulmonary function testing, and other requirements, depending on institutional policy. Some PAPR units are noisy enough to warrant participation in hearing conservation programs as well.

Gloves used for HLCC protect the health care worker's hands from

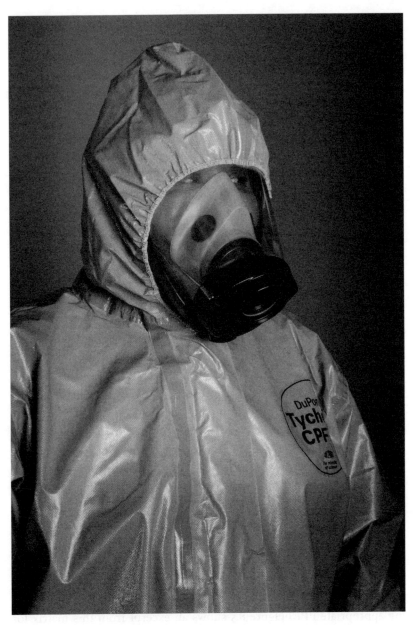

Figure 8.4. Full-Facepiece Respirator (Courtesy of Nebraska Medicine)

body fluids and chemicals such as cleaning solutions. Disposable gloves manufactured from nitrile, neoprene, or other nonlatex materials are less likely to cause skin and respiratory reactions than natural rubber latex. Long-cuff nitrile gloves provide extended coverage for the wrist and lower arm and reduce the risk of separation from the sleeve cuff of a gown or suit. Reusable gloves (e.g. thick, chemical-resistant nitrile) are best reserved for nonpatient care duties, as they tend to be less form fitting and more difficult to use when fine motor skills are needed.

Body coverings include scrubs, gowns, aprons, coveralls, footwear, and boot covers. Materials can be fluid resistant or impermeable and single-use or reusable. Reusable items can lose some of their durability and effectiveness during the decontamination and laundering processes. Although some expert panels advocate fluid-impermeable materials for enhanced contact precautions for VHF, fluid-resistant materials are adequate for some applications and can be combined with fluid-impermeable aprons or other equipment when high-volume fluid exposure may be expected. Special attention should be given to gown and suit seams, however, because unsealed stitched seams can provide a direct portal of entry. Scrubs worn as a base layer of PPE should be loose fitting and comfortable and do not necessarily need to be fluid resistant. When selecting gowns, aprons, coveralls, and boot covers, consider products that provide protection based on transmission risk. Coveralls should be worn loosely to allow the suit to easily roll over the shoulders when doffing, and to reduce the likelihood of a seam breach. PPE selection should account for the clinical challenges presented by basic patient care and interaction, close contact with large amounts of body fluids, aerosol generating procedures, and even postmortem care. Procedures outside of patient care areas, such as waste processing and equipment disinfection, may also require special protective equipment relative to the nature of the hazards present and the work to be done.

OSHA published a PPE selection matrix for protection against occupational exposure to Ebola to assist employers in identifying and selecting appropriate PPE. Figure 8.5 shows an excerpt from this matrix for individuals that provide medical and supportive care for patients being screened or treated for EVD.

Approach to Donning and Doffing. While PPE can effectively protect

Table 8.1. Checklist for Donning and Doffing with a Disposable Respirator. Adapted from Beam et al. (2015). Used with permission.

Donning Checklist	Doffing Checklist
1. Boot covers	1. Tape
2. Surgical hood	2. Long-cuff gloves secured with duct tape
3. Gown	
4. Disposable respirator (N95 or P100) and seal check	3. Doffing partner change gloves
	4. Gown
5. Face shield	5. Inner gloves
6. Hand hygiene	6. Doffing partner and doffer change gloves
7. Exam gloves	
8. Long-cuff gloves secured with duct tape	7. Face shield
	8. Disposable respirator (N95 or P100)
9. Safety check	
10. Third layer of gloves, aprons for patient care	9. Surgical hood
	10. Bleach wipe plastic footwear
	11. Hand hygiene
	12. Antimicrobial wipe personal eyewear
	13. Shower

HCW from exposure and transmission, it only works when used appropriately. Human factors often limit PPE effectiveness, such as forgetting to secure ties on an isolation gown or touching the filter surface of a respirator during removal. Complete compliance with PPE protocols for donning and doffing should not rely on memory alone. Most units use a variety of donning and doffing aids, including posted checklists, picture references, buddy checks, and external observers to confirm proper sequence and actions and thus reduce the likelihood of human errors leading to contamination. Tables 8.1 and 8.2 provide examples of checklists employed in our biocontainment unit. Other interventions to reduce human error include full-length mirrors to allow self-checks of donned PPE and video recording of donning and doffing procedures to

Table 8.2. Checklist for Donning and Doffing with a PAPR. Adapted from Beam et al. (2015). Used with permission.

Donning Checklist	Doffing Checklist
1. Boot liners	1. Tape
2. Protective suit to waist	2. Long-cuff gloves
3. Boot covers	3. Boot covers
4. Exam gloves	4. PAPR belt
5. Suit to upper body	5. Protective suit
6. PAPR belt with blower and tubing	6. Exam gloves: replace with clean gloves
7. Long-cuff gloves secured with duct tape	7. Switch PAPR off
8. Attach tubing to PAPR hood	8. Undo PAPR tubing from the motor
9. Turn on the blower and put on hood	9. Place filter cap on PAPR motor
10. Tuck inner collar into suit	10. PAPR hood
11. Zip suit to neck and seal flap	11. Boot liners
12. Lay outer collar over suit	12. Bleach wipe plastic footwear
13. Safety check	13. Hand hygiene, clean gloves
14. Third layer of gloves, aprons for patient care	14. Antimicrobial wipe personal eyewear
	15. Shower

allow for systematic assessment. As with most critical human activities, simplicity and repeatability are important themes in developing donning and doffing protocols.

Donning Procedures. The process of donning PPE occurs in a controlled environment outside of the at-risk zone but requires training with equal vigilance to detail as with doffing. Individuals should remove jewelry and personal items (e.g., watches, earrings, pens, cell phones) before starting the donning process, and the unit should provide safe storage options to incentivize behavior. Donning sequence will vary depending on equipment used in the PPE ensemble, but it should be specified well in advance by organizational leadership and workers trained on a regular basis. As donning sequence frequently drives doffing sequence, donning protocols should account for core principles and priorities in doffing, namely, removing the most contaminated items first, maintaining protection of the eyes and respiratory tract for as long as possible, and facilitating appropriate hand hygiene.

Gowns are worn with the opening to the back of the body and secured at the neck and waist. Eye and face protection should be secured behind the ears or over the head. Donning order for gloves will depend on the level of protection needed. If more than one layer of gloves is used, the final layer should overlap the cuffs on the gown's sleeves. Some HLCC unit protocols also use tape at the interface of the glove and sleeve to prevent unintentional skin exposure. This is an institutional preference but when done should use tape that does not tear sleeve material with removal and should incorporate a folded-over tab to enable ease of removal and to prevent tears.

When used, a respirator is placed over the nose, mouth, and chin, then secured to the head with elastic straps and adjusted to fit. A seal check is performed after the respirator is situated firmly against the face; the respirator should collapse in toward the face during inhalation. During exhalation, air should exit through the respirator (or valve) and not escape around the sides. A general principle for tight-fitting respirators is that equipment that is in place before donning the respirator should not impede direct contact of the mask and straps with the wearer's head. Straps that secure the respirator in place should not be placed over goggles or another eye protection and should be used per design (i.e., no cross-strapping). The PAPR provides a loose-fitting alternative for respiratory protection that also protects the eyes. Before donning a PAPR, complete a safety check of the blower, battery, and air supply hose. PAPRs vary by manufacturer and should be donned according to the manufacturer's guidelines.

Doffing Procedures. The doffing procedure depends greatly on the layout and design of the specific HLCC unit. Regardless, doffing should consist of a coordinated sequence that removes potential sources of contamination while moving stepwise from areas of higher to lower contamination risk. While zones of risk are best separated by physical barriers (walls and doors), simple distance with tape lines or other demarcation may suffice. Doffing begins prior to exit from the high-risk zone. Before removing any PPE, the wearer and the doffing partner should inspect PPE for tears or other breaches in the integrity of the material, disinfect any areas of visible or suspected contamination, and identify areas that are considered contaminated and clean. In general, the most contaminated areas are the front of the PPE ensemble, gloves, and sleeves—where there was a likelihood of coming into contact with the patient or the environment. Generally, areas of PPE that are considered cleaner are the back side of the PPE ensemble, where it is less likely that the PPE came in contact with the patient or the environment.

The doffing sequence depends on the equipment used and the order that it was donned. When multiple layers of gloves are used, the outermost that had frequent contact with patients or contaminated environments can be decontaminated and removed prior to leaving the patient care area. A new outer glove may be donned, if necessary, to ensure that at least two pairs of gloves are present to initiate the formal doffing sequence. In addition, some units will also remove an outer apron or gown inside the patient care area in order to contain materials with the highest likelihood and degree of contamination inside the high-risk zone. If conducted in the patient care area, these actions should occur as far away from areas of intense contamination (such as the patient) as possible and close to the exit, to limit opportunities for further contamination prior to leaving the highest-risk zone. The use of chemical sprayers, foot baths, and wipes for decontamination in doffing is a point of debate and remains an institutional decision. Selection of doffing decontamination methods should account for the environment considerations (indoors, outdoors, drains) when selecting an appropriate method. Some experts have expressed concern regarding the opportunity for splash and re-aerosolization associated with decontamination sprayers in enclosed spaces. Since most HLCC units in developed countries operate in fixed indoor facilities with finished flooring, sprayers may create slip and chemical fume hazards for HCWs and patients that may be more consequential. Disinfectant wipe options do exist for decontamination beyond gross soiling (which is universally recommended) and in high-risk scenarios may provide an extra margin of safety.

As doffing proceeds, PPE on the body should be removed prior to

PPE protecting the head and face. This provides mucous membrane protection from any aerosolization that might occur as contaminated PPE on the body is removed. When drafting and training doffing procedures, the mantra "Clean touches clean; dirty touches dirty" can help reinforce principles for avoiding cross contamination. External gloves (considered more dirty) should touch external surfaces of gowns and suits, while inside surfaces of PPE garments and inner-layer gloves (all considered more clean) should touch each other. Assistance from a doffing partner or a chair or stool can reduce the fall risk associated with balance issues and fatigue. When removing gloves, the wearer should use the glove-in-glove technique, creating a bundle of both gloves, with the least contaminated surfaces on the outside, that is gently discarded. After each doffing step in which the wearer touches a component of PPE, hand hygiene with alcohol-based hand rub or handwashing should be performed. When removing a gown, a doffing partner can carefully unfasten ties at the neck and waste, which reduces opportunity for aerosol generation or splatter when these ties are forcibly torn. Doffing partners can also help with zippers on suits. Removal of gowns, suits, and boot or shoe covers while avoiding cross contamination is one of the more challenging aspects of doffing. Specific procedures should account for the style and model of garment being removed and for dexterity challenges associated with staff fatigue. Doffing partners and rolling techniques (to contain outer dirty layers and expose clean inner surfaces) can be employed to reduce risk of self-contamination. Handles, chairs, or stools can help provide balance and support to prevent falls and stumbles.

Core principles of safety during doffing include slow and intentional movements, control of garments to avoid flailing of dragging pieces, diligent attention to hand hygiene, and protection of mucous membranes. The doffing process is significantly aided by visual cues from the observer/doffing partner or marked on floors or walls. Sensible placement of waste receptacles and hand hygiene stations can greatly streamline the process. Trash cans with larger mouth openings make easier targets for disposing doffed garments and may reduce the urge to push down trash, which presents a re-aerosolization hazard.

The last stage of doffing is hand hygiene performed outside the area of risk and removal of scrubs and other clothing that was worn under

PPE in the patient care area. Some units require staff to "shower out" of the unit, taking a personal shower after removing scrubs. While not necessary for most situations, it may be advisable for certain high-risk scenarios and can simply provide peace of mind to the personnel providing HLCC.

Disinfection

Disinfection is the process of destroying, or rendering inactive, biological pathogens by physical or chemical means. Although technically different terms, disinfection and decontamination are often used interchangeably within the HLCC environment. Disinfection should be conducted frequently during HLCC operations. Spot disinfection is used in instances where visible contamination is present, such as body fluid spills. Daily disinfection involves routine cleaning with appropriate disinfectants to reduce pathogen load on surfaces. Terminal decontamination is the final definitive process to remove pathogen contamination after patient care operations cease. Disinfection should be conducted by trained professionals utilizing the proper PPE, taking into account the causal microorganism, disinfectant(s), and the environmental conditions. In HLCC operations, HCWs can be cross-trained to conduct spot and daily disinfection as functions of routine duties. This can be beneficial as it reduces the number of individuals who come into the HLCC unit and are subject to risk.

The causal microorganism will drive the disinfectant selection. In the United States, the EPA has authority on the registering of disinfectants, and only EPA-registered hospital disinfectants with a label claim for the particular pathogen should be utilized. In a case where such a label claim does not exist, seek guidance from both the US EPA and CDC prior to deciding on disinfection technique, as was done during the 2014–16 West Africa EVD outbreak.

When utilizing a disinfectant, it is critical that the manufacturer's instructions be followed for its proper use, particularly around minimum contact times and concentration. Many chemical disinfectants lose potency when exposed to oxygen, high temperatures, and humidity; therefore, staff should monitor the expiration time/date or age of each compound both before and after they are prepared for use. Because the organic load of gross contamination (e.g., blood, feces, other body fluids, etc.) will drastically reduce the efficacy of any disinfectant, gross contamination must be mechanically removed prior to disinfection. The HLCC environment may present scenarios not covered by the manufacturer's instructions, and in these cases it is recommended that you consult with the proper professionals, including representatives from the US EPA and CDC. If the causal microorganism is unknown, then often the disinfectant utilized should be a more robust disinfectant with a US EPA–registered hospital disinfectant with a label claim against spores, such as the US EPA List K disinfectants.

An effective daily cleaning/disinfection routine should be established and maintained throughout HLCC operations; however, staff should take advantage of every opportunity to clean and disinfect throughout the day. As with other movement in HLCC units, cleaning should proceed from the least contaminated (cold) zone to the most contaminated (hot) zones, ideally with each zone having its own designated cleaning and disinfecting equipment.

Several options exist for whole room disinfection associated with terminal cleaning and decontamination (e.g., UVGI, gaseous chlorine dioxide, and vaporized hydrogen peroxide). Whole room disinfection should occur after patient discharge and should be performed by personnel specifically trained in how to do so safely, including proper PPE selection and use. Environmental science and industrial hygiene experts should weigh whole room disinfectant options for each facility accounting for specific needs. For example, UVGI is effective at surface disinfection but requires that the UV light reach all surfaces for the proper amount of exposure. This method would be less effective in rooms crowded with equipment or with hidden and shielded areas.

Movement of Waste and Materials Out of Containment

Design and operation of HLCC units should account for movement of waste and other materials (e.g., patient specimens) out of HLCC settings. Waste management constitutes one of the more challenging features of HLCC and is covered extensively in chapter 19. However, principles pertaining to design and protocol for movement of materials out of containment will be addressed here.

As a general rule, materials exiting the unit are either rendered non-infectious prior to passing out of the unit or are sealed in redundant layers of protective containment. All surfaces—bags and containers—are extensively decontaminated with appropriate disinfectant wipes or sprays. The authors prefer to pass out or receive materials in rigid containers in order to reduce the odds of plastic bag tears or punctures that could result in breach of containment. Air locks or pass-through boxes (with interlocking doors) provide the highest safety margin for passing material out of the isolation space; however, these features are expensive to retrofit and infrequently featured in patient units. Pass-through boxes can be fitted with UV irradiators to provide additional safety. While pass-through dunk tanks also offer a high degree of protection from cross contamination, we do not recommend their use in HLCC due to associated splash and slip hazards. In most instances, materials are passed out of a briefly opened door and to a receiving person outside of isolation who is wearing appropriate PPE, depending on the material and pathogen involved. For most pathogens with limited aerosol transmission potential (e.g., viral hemorrhagic fever viruses) opening a door from a lower risk (warm) area to the cold zone presents negligible risk of pathogen escape, primarily due to the negative pressure gradient that exists. However, for small spaces without antechambers and with airborne pathogens, this risk may be more substantial. Ideally, solid waste materials are decontaminated prior to removal from the containment space, which reduces requirements for further safe handling and hazardous materials shipping and disposal procedures.

Lab specimens to be passed out of isolation can be sealed in at least two layers of leak-proof bags that are surface decontaminated (with contact time necessary to achieve decontamination) and then passed out by one of the above methods to the outside of the HLCC unit for transportation to the laboratory for analysis. Sample seals should be maintained and not opened until they are within the containment of a biological safety cabinet within the laboratory. Passage of all other materials, supplies, and equipment that cannot be autoclaved can be sent out through air locks/fumigation chambers where they are subjected to chemical gas disinfection, or another approved process (e.g., disinfection and desiccation), prior to removal.

HLCC Unit Leadership, Staffing, and Training

Unit Leadership. An interprofessional leadership team to provide strategic direction is critical to HLCC readiness and operational success. Such a team should integrate nurse leaders, physicians, biosafety and infection control professionals, laboratorians, and industrial hygienists. The leadership team must embrace a mindset and culture of safety. Additionally, in the complex environment of HLCC, a comprehensive approach to problem-solving and decision-making, pursuit of novel ideas, and adherence to evidence-based protocols can dramatically improve team performance. The leadership team should meet frequently to discuss key components of biocontainment unit operations: research, protocols, emergency response, staff engagement, training and exercise plans, and progress.

Staff Recruitment and Selection. Biocontainment unit staffing must take into account the facility's organizational structure, physical layout, institutional staffing requirements (for noncontainment wards), and organized labor (union) considerations. Currently in the United States, some Ebola treatment centers (ETCs) include HLCC duties as a component of standard hospital job descriptions. For unionized labor, this approach provides the foundation for contractual agreements that include HLCC care. When it is a tenable strategy, volunteer-based staffing allows for a more selective process and more buy-in from staff.

Ultimately, the HLCC staff must possess a solid foundation of clinical skills and sufficient expertise to manage complex patients, often critically ill, in a challenging environment. Because the appropriate care of the patient with an HHCD and the risk of pathogen transmission to staff must constantly drive decisions, infectious disease physician involvement is central. Critical care nurses and physicians form an important core of the health care team in HLCC, but staff from wards, emergency departments, and other backgrounds bring important diversity of perspective and problem-solving. Staff should also include other skilled professions required for care and safe operations such as respiratory therapists, infection prevention specialists, industrial hygienists, environmental scientists, and so on. Other skilled positions such as imaging and dialysis technicians can be fully incorporated into the team or may be able to cross-train and guide unit staff to be able to manage specific applications. Due to the challenges and stress of HLCC operations, staff should have preexisting experience in their care discipline and must possess critical thinking skills, work well on a team, embrace strong attention to detail, and demonstrate psychological stability. These characteristics can be assessed by using a standardized psychological assessment tool.

Onboarding. Once selected, team members should undergo a structured onboarding process to include orientation and initial training. Onboarding should focus on skills and equipment unique to the HLCC environment. Key areas to consider include safe entry and exit procedures, modified patient assessment techniques, waste management, decedent management, body fluid management, and donning and doffing procedures for selected PPE. Emergency response plans should also be communicated to new incoming staff. Introductory educational modules should be tailored to include discipline-specific considerations when including physicians, nurses, respiratory therapists, or other support staff. Onboarding should allow for ample time, training, and supervised work prior to certification for independent operations within the HLCC environment.

Routine Training. Standardized training should be coordinated by a structured training program that establishes requirements for initial certification of competency in independent biocontainment work and specific tasks designated for general personnel and specific specialty. The training program should track up-to-date relevance and provide training plans to maintain currency and individual certification for HLCC operations. Although no national or international standards exist at this time, we recommend training at least annually for all facilities and at least quarterly in designated regional ETCs by rostered staff members. At a minimum, training should include donning and doffing of PPE, review of protocols that address high-impact, low-frequency events such as "provider down" and decedent management, and performance of basic skills. Units should develop an evaluation process that addresses both individual proficiency and team dynamics. The ability to evaluate and trend both individual and team progress over time will assist with the progressive enhancement of a training program that meets the needs of the rostered staff. In addition, it is critical that a method be determined to accurately track the attendance and performance of all HLCC team members. This documentation can be used to guide any just-in-time (JIT) training material development and deployment if the biocontainment unit is activated.

In addition to routine training, implementing a progressive multiyear training and exercise plan that adheres to Homeland Security Exercise and Evaluation Program (HSEEP) guidance will serve to continually advance HLCC capabilities. HLCC staff should be encouraged to participate on the exercise planning committee. Inviting team members to participate in exercise planning procedures provides a strategy to foster development of additional expertise, a deeper knowledge of HLCC unit operations and SOPs, and team engagement. Incorporating a variety of discussion-based and operational exercises provides staff members and leadership with a venue to test the SOPs that have been established and make any necessary improvements. At a minimum these exercises should consider activation, transportation, admission, and patient care procedures. When structuring a training and exercise program for HLCC teams, it is advisable to start with basic, plausible scenarios. This allows the leadership team to fine tune protocols and establish a foundation of trust and confidence within the team. As the team progresses, exercises can be expanded to include specialized scenarios such as surgical interventions and multiple patient admissions. Incorporating emergency management experts in constructing exercises can also optimize support and assist with meeting essential exercise requirements.

Just-in-Time Training. Health care professionals that are not included among the rostered HLCC staff but whose expertise may be needed should have access to JIT training prior to providing care in the HLCC unit. However, completion of JIT training should not be interpreted as having the HLCC facility knowledge and skills to operate autonomously but should prepare the trainee to enter the environment under direct supervision of HLCC staff. A JIT training curriculum should include essential elements that are critical to safe patient care delivery, identified by a risk assessment of potential tasks to be carried out. Focal areas to consider include safe entry and exit procedures, PPE donning and doffing, role-specific procedures to be performed in PPE, and communication techniques in the hot zone. Delivery methods should be tailored to the needs of the individual and include multiple strategies such as online modules, electronic distribution, and in-person hands-on training.

Resilience Training. The incorporation of resilience and mindfulness strategies into routine training for HLCC team members should be considered an essential component of a comprehensive training and exercise plan. HLCC units providing patient care have cited mental health as an important element in a biocontainment unit occupational health program. HCWs who provided care for patients in the Nebraska Biocontainment Unit known to have EVD identified interpersonal stressors to include alterations in their home or social life or feeling isolated during the period of activation. Integrating behavioral health experts into the HLCC team training provides easy access to rostered staff and helps instill healthy coping mechanisms in team members. Having a behavioral health worker available for staff members during training helps foster strong relationships in advance of an actual event. Several HLCC-activated staff identified that having a behavioral health expert available for informal conversations was beneficial during activations. Strategies to enhance the focus on resiliency include team training events, inclusion of presentations and time to practice techniques before or after drills and exercises, and inviting behavioral health experts to observe and participate in scheduled trainings.

HLCC Team Culture

Effective HLCC operations require a unique team culture of cohesion, communication, teamwork, problem-solving, and above all safety. Safety must permeate all day-to-day activities, training, and operations. Leadership must embrace this concept and act deliberately toward that goal. Ideally, each team meeting or function should begin and end with a safety message, and safety concerns should be the ultimate point of emphasis before entry into the HLCC unit.

A horizontal hierarchy is one key component of this culture, where each staff member feels empowered to speak up to address safety issues.

Because staffing inside the biocontainment unit is at a premium, custodial tasks and scut work must be performed by all individuals within the unit, from the medical director to the newest technician. The philosophy that nobody is above any job begins to build a culture of shared responsibility. Staff members should be trained to leave rank and title at the door of the HLCC unit, and teams can consider using first names in addressing each other within HLCC.

A team with horizontal hierarchy, where every member feels they have equal value, importance, and responsibility for safe operations, will manage unexpected hazards more effectively. Every HLCC unit should have a code word that informs team members of a safety concern and immediately prompts them to stop all activity and listen. Often this code word is as simple as "STOP!" In a team with appropriate safety culture, every member would feel empowered and obligated to call a time-out as soon as they encounter a major safety concern. On hearing the code word, all team members should cease movement (or proceed to the first safe stopping point), listen to the concern (described in direct and succinct terms) from the member who raised the alarm, and jointly formulate a plan to address the hazard. This concept should be taught and drilled constantly to become second nature.

Conclusion

Safe and effective operation in HLCC requires an efficient and high-functioning unit, working in accordance with foundational principles of containment care. HLCC operations rely heavily on implementation of the HoC. Most importantly, they rely on meticulous planning, tested SOPs, and continuous training of staff. A highly functioning HLCC unit and team requires a significant commitment of time and resources.

While no national or international certifying body exists for HLCC, and practice will necessarily vary among different units related to unique features, most aforementioned engineering controls are not only practice- and evidence-based but also validated through analysis. Thus, consensus design and engineering features among high-level isolation units in developed nations should be considered the "gold standard" for engineering controls in HLCC units. In addition, a growing evidence base supports some consensus practice in administrative controls and PPE. With continued research, best practices can be established across all components of HLCC operations.

Adherence to the infection control and biocontainment practices in HLCC units implemented by interdisciplinary teams with competency in patient care, biosafety, infection control, and utilization of PPE will allow your organization to establish a facility and operations to safely care for these unique patients. While there are many different ways to accomplish these goals, the basic principles of safety continue to apply. Mindfulness toward the mental well-being of all those involved will also contribute toward the success of your HLCC unit.

CHAPTER 9

Patient Care in High-Level Containment Care Units

In a Resourced Setting

ANGELA M. VASA
KATE C. BOULTER
JOLENE M. HORIHAN
DAVID S. CATES
CRAIG A. PIQUETTE
JAMES N. SULLIVAN
DANIEL W. JOHNSON
ANGELA L. HEWLETT

An Introduction to the Delivery of Care in Personal Protective Equipment

The ability of experienced clinicians to provide safe care in a high-level containment care (HLCC) unit can be impacted when wearing the advanced personal protective equipment (PPE) that is required when treating individuals with highly hazardous communicable diseases (HHCDs). Caregivers must be aware of the effect that wearing this level of PPE can have on the senses, their ability to communicate effectively, and their inability to sustain their efforts over time as compared to without PPE. Noise from negative air pressure ventilation systems in the care environment and the use of powered air-purifying respirators (PAPR) may diminish auditory abilities. Visual perception may also be diminished by the limited visual fields of visors, goggles, and face shields. Fine motor skills and tactile sensation may be impeded by the use of two or three layers of gloves. In addition, physical endurance while wearing PPE for an extended period of time may be diminished and varies by health care worker. It is dependent on several factors: baseline level of conditioning, the level of energy expended while in PPE, the individual's threshold for heat tolerance, and any underlying illnesses. Due to these factors, it is desirable that clinicians who will be expected to provide care for patients in the HLCC unit have advanced training that includes performing activities appropriate for their role and skills while wearing PPE. In the event standardized training is not completed prior to an actual event, just-in-time (JIT) training should be provided prior to entering the patient care area to ensure that care providers continue to have some baseline understanding of the challenges of working in PPE.

Clinicians should be instructed on modifications to usual practice that may be required when performing standard patient assessments within the HLCC unit. Access to customary equipment, including stethoscopes, otoscopes, or other devices, may be limited due to infection prevention concerns and the challenges of using such equipment while wearing PPE. The inability to auscultate heart and lung sounds routinely is one of the significant challenges identified by nurses and physicians who have practiced in an HLCC setting. Adjusting assessment techniques to accommodate these restrictions requires flexibility and innovative thinking.

Various adaptive devices are available that can be used to enhance the level of care provided in HLCC units, each with its own unique features and challenges. Electronic and digital stethoscopes with Bluetooth technology have advantages that include sound amplification, the ability to adjust the listening frequency, and the potential use of disposable headphones and headsets for auscultation, allowing the clinician to insert the devices into their ear canals prior to entry into the unit. Disadvantages include increased cost and the need for access to electricity or replacement batteries for charging. Bluetooth stethoscopes may have broadcasting interference, and electronic stethoscopes may be susceptible to electronic interference by other devices. In addition to the use of specialized auscultation instruments, telehealth equipment can be incorporated to augment head-to-toe assessments. Otoscopes and ophthalmoscopes can be added as options to many telehealth platforms, which allow providers to complete detailed assessments from the "cold" zone of the HLCC unit. This is key to limiting the footprint in the contaminated "hot" zone as much as possible while still providing a standard of care commensurate with or exceeding that in the general inpatient wards.

Telehealth can be a significant component in operating an HLCC unit. In addition to enhancing assessment capabilities, it bridges a note-worthy communication gap. Telehealth products can allow the health care staff to communicate with the patient from the clean area using both audio and video technology to enrich communication. Telehealth products can also be used to allow the patient to communicate with their identified support system, including family and friends. In an isolation care setting all efforts should be made to allow the patient to communicate safely and freely with their loved ones.

The addition of any technology can mitigate some of the challenges encountered when wearing advanced PPE, but the inclusion of these devices for HLCC must include a risk assessment that weighs the potential advantages and barriers of including the equipment.

Staffing

Nursing Staffing. Identifying team members to provide care in the HLCC setting may present a unique challenge in recruitment due to the perceived risk of working in such a unit. The ability to discern appropriate staff is a quality that should be inherent in the leadership team tasked with creating the staff roster. When determining the minimum standards for job descriptions for HLCC staff, a number of factors should be considered: the size of the overall nursing support staff available in the facility; the type of care expected to be provided in the HLCC unit; the demographics of patients to be admitted; the number of beds available in the HLCC unit; and the availability of additional support staff who can augment the nursing team. These are all essential components to address when designing a strategy to staff an advanced isolation care area. Once the core team is established, nurse leaders should create a staffing matrix that will guide unit operations during an activation. One consideration in this approach is that there must be flexibility built into the process to account for rapid changes in patient acuity, staff endurance in PPE, and staff availability.

Staffing for the admission of a patient with a pathogen that warrants HLCC differs greatly from staffing a standard inpatient unit. In general, the designated HLCC units across the United States rely on a majority of staff who are otherwise employed in departments elsewhere within the facility. This staffing model requires that nurse managers or program directors implement an on-call or "ghost" schedule to identify staff who are available to respond to an activation at any given time. In addition to maintaining a ready roster of staff, the staffing ratios in an HLCC unit require more resource-heavy models. In a typical intensive care unit, the standard ratio is one nurse to two critically ill patients; in an HLCC setting, US models for a patient admitted with a viral hemorrhagic fever (VHF) can be closer to three nurses to one patient for a 12-hour shift. In addition to these 3 nurses, who are responsible for providing direct patient care, an additional 2 to 3 staff members per shift are included on the schedule to support other activities within the unit, bringing the overall ratio for staff to an average of 5–6 for a census of one patient. An increase in census will create the need for an increase in staff assigned to the care of the patients. As with any patient, the minimum number of staff needed for the team will vary depending on the acuity level of the patients and whether more than one nurse is required to remain at the bedside. This approach to staffing is necessary to account for the various roles needed to maintain function of a closed unit and to accommodate modified shift times due to the limited amount of time that care providers can remain in PPE. The model used in the Nebraska Biocontainment Unit (NBU) incorporates key roles and their designated functions into standard operation procedures (SOPs) that are part of the operational protocols, which include the primary nurse, task nurse, front desk nurse, doffing partner, autoclave operator, and tasker (see table 9.1). Each of these roles rotates in 4-hour increments during a standard 12-hour shift.

Table 9.1 Examples of Staff Roles in a Biocontainment Unit

Primary nurse—registered nurse who serves as the coordinator of patient care between the nurses on each shift, ensuring that all nursing duties and charting requirements are fulfilled.

Task nurse—registered nurse who serves as the liaison at the front desk to assist the nurse in the patient care area in executing needed tasks and physicians' orders.

Front desk nurse/trained observer—registered nurse who answers the phones, coordinates with physicians, and monitors the audio/visual feed from the hot zone in order to ensure adherence to infection prevention and control principles.

Doffing partner—rostered staff member who remains in the warm zone and serves a dual purpose by assisting the care providers exiting the care area with doffing PPE and acting as a courier between the cold zone and the hot zone. This person is in the same level of PPE as the provider in the patient care area and, in the event that additional assistance is needed in the patient care area, can quickly and safely enter the room.

Autoclave operator—rostered staff member who receives the waste from the hot zone and processes it through the autoclave. This team member is donned in PPE that is appropriate for the level of risk associated with the waste being processed.

Tasker—rostered staff member who coordinates communication and acquisition of supplies, serves as the liaison with incident command, and provides coverage for the front desk nurse/trained observer during breaks.

This approach allows care providers wearing the required PPE in the patient care areas to switch out in order to limit heat stress and fatigue.

Physician Staffing. Caring for patients with HHCDs requires a multidisciplinary physician team. In the HLCC setting, physician leaders may include infectious disease as well as critical care specialists. Infectious disease specialists manage antimicrobial therapy, monitor viral loads and other markers of infection, evaluate for secondary infectious processes, and oversee the administration of experimental therapeutic agents. Critical care medicine specialists are an important part of the physician team, since patients with HHCDs are often critically ill and may require mechanical ventilation, vasopressors, and invasive procedures. HLCC units may have different specialists in charge, depending on local preference, needs, and availability.

Other physicians, including those who care for special populations, should be included on the physician team. Recruitment efforts for HLCC units that have the potential to care for pediatric patients should include pediatricians and pediatric intensive care specialists. Obstetricians should also be part of the physician team, in case a pregnant woman and/or patient in labor may require care in the HLCC unit. Nephrology specialists may be needed to care for patients with HHCDs, especially those with VHFs, who may develop acute renal failure and require dialysis. Relationships should be established with other physician groups, including surgery, pathology, and emergency medicine, since consultations (either in-person or via telemedicine) may become necessary.

Physicians providing care to patients in an HLCC unit may be unavailable to care for other patients in the hospital/clinic for prolonged periods, so it is important to consider having a backfilling plan for other clinical responsibilities. There is a consensus among many HLCC unit leaders that clinicians in training (fellows, residents, students) should not provide direct care for patients with HHCDs due to excessive risk and the desire to limit the number of individuals entering the patient room. Clinicians in training may be able to participate, observe, and assist with the management of patients remotely or via a telemedicine system.

Cohorting. The decision to cohort patients in the HLCC setting is dependent on several factors, including the number of patients requiring care, the physical structure and capabilities of the HLCC unit, the availability of an adequate number of staff, the clinical characteristics of the disease, the equipment needs of the patient, and many others. The medical director should make any decisions about cohorting in consultation with a multidisciplinary leadership team to ensure that all factors are considered. If the decision is made to cohort individuals in an HLCC unit, attention must be paid to infection prevention and control measures. HLCC unit staff should receive JIT training on how to modify SOPs to include strategies to minimize cross contamination between patients. Every effort should be made to maintain the privacy and dignity of those individuals who are being placed in a semiprivate environment in an HLCC setting.

Bedside Procedures

Medical procedures should be performed at the bedside in the HLCC unit whenever possible, since transporting patients infected with HHCDs to other locations may introduce significant risk of contamination of the hospital facility, as well as potential transmission to others. When considering the provision of bedside procedures in the HLCC unit, it is critical to ensure that experienced physicians are available to perform these procedures. Procedural skills can be assessed by direct consultation with these physicians, since some may not feel comfortable performing invasive procedures in an HLCC setting. Training and drills involving the performance of invasive procedures while in PPE should be part of routine training and preparedness for physicians who will be tasked with performing these procedures in the HLCC unit.

Invasive procedures pose an increased risk to the patient and operator any time they are performed. This is especially true in the HLCC setting when the operator is wearing enhanced PPE and treating patients with HHCDs. PPE can make procedures difficult by limiting visibility, decreasing tactile sensation, and preventing the movement of air and heat from the body, making fog and perspiration major issues. Although many of these procedures are performed alone in standard care environments, it is recommended to have an assistant available in the HLCC environment to increase the safety and efficiency of the procedure. It is critical that the operator and assistant discuss the details and planned sequence of the procedure beforehand. Individuals performing high-risk procedures in high-level isolation environments should consider the use of PAPRs in order to decrease the risk of exposure. However, wearing PAPRs could impair the ability to communicate effectively and could cause eye irritation from the air blowing inside the hood; therefore, the decision on the specific PPE should be based on risk assessment.

Vascular Access. Central venous catheters (CVCs) are necessary to deliver fluid resuscitation, medications, and total parenteral nutrition to critically ill patients. Ultrasound guidance should be utilized, and operators with extensive experience in CVC placement should perform the procedure. In the HLCC unit, it may be necessary to leave a CVC in place longer than the standard practice in order to decrease the risk of a needle stick exposure by eliminating the need for traditional phlebotomy. CVCs should be placed in the left internal jugular vein using ultrasound guidance, leaving the right internal jugular site available for hemodialysis access if needed. The catheter should be secured to the skin with sutureless adhesive dressings to reduce the chance of needle sticks. Ultrasonography may be used to evaluate for the presence of a pneumothorax and confirm appropriate placement if the operator is experienced in this technique. Alternatively, conventional chest radiographs can be used if available. CVC sites should be monitored frequently for signs of infection, and the site should be maintained with strict attention to infection control practices. Peripherally inserted central catheters (PICCs) may be considered, but placement of a PICC line may be extremely difficult in patients who are severely volume depleted. The use of arterial catheters to monitor blood pressure and obtain arterial blood gases can also be considered for critically ill patients in HLCC settings.

Airway Management. In HLCC settings, it is reasonable to perform elective intubation in patients who have early manifestations of respiratory compromise in order to avoid emergency intubation scenarios. Airway management should be performed by experienced operators due to the increased risk in this setting. Since intubation presents a significant risk of aerosolization, PAPRs should be worn in order to provide the best protection. Rapid sequence induction including neuromuscular blockade while utilizing video laryngoscopy is recommended to reduce the likelihood of exposure to the operator.

Prior to performing intubation in the HLCC setting, staffing should be optimized to include an experienced intensive care nurse or critical care respiratory therapist in the room. In addition to the standard safety measures, if patient condition allows it is helpful to walk through the entire procedure in advance of executing intubation. This helps ensure that all staff are clear on their roles and expectations for assisting in a successful and safe intubation.

Dialysis. Patients admitted to an HLCC unit may require continuous renal replacement therapy (CRRT), or dialysis in severe cases, to manage renal failure and electrolyte disturbances. CRRT is an intervention routinely used in intensive care units to support patients with acute renal failure. The aims of RRT are solute and water removal, correction of electrolyte abnormalities, and normalization of acid-base disturbances. The benefit to considering the use of CRRT as an alternative approach to conventional hemodialysis in an HLCC unit is that it can be successfully managed at the bedside by critical care nurses and telehealth consultation with nephrologists. Advocates of continuous therapy compared to intermittent techniques claim that there is enhanced hemodynamic stability, superior management of fluid balance, and enhanced clearance of inflammatory mediators. As with any type of hemodialysis, patients in an HLCC unit will require the insertion of a hemodialysis line to enable timely initiation of hemodialysis. As patients with HHCDs may experience large fluid shifts and resultant electrolyte imbalances, planning for the provision of hemodialysis should be considered when creating SOPs and recruiting staff for HLCC units. Similar to what is noted above, appropriate PPE will be needed for central venous access and during aspects of dialysis that may involve potential exposures to blood or body fluids. Because a significant minority of patients with severe VHF manifestations may need renal salvage, HLCC units should ensure appropriate coverage or a method for JIT training for a nephrologist and dialysis technicians.

Other Procedures. Thoracentesis, paracentesis, or lumbar puncture may be required either for diagnostic or therapeutic reasons. As with any invasive procedures, a risk assessment should be completed in advance of implementing any interventions and appropriate PPE worn. It has become standard of care to utilize ultrasound guidance in the performance of many invasive bedside procedures, and when feasible, operators experienced in using ultrasound guidance should be involved.

Bedside Surgery vs. Transport to the Operating Theater. Although it is desirable to perform all procedures at the bedside in the HLCC unit, consideration may be given to the transport of HLCC patients on a case-by-case basis. A careful risk-benefit assessment should be conducted, and should include disease-specific transmission risk, the clinical status of the patient, the urgency of the need for surgical intervention, and the training of the surgical team. These factors should be weighed against the risks to the facility, health care workers, and other patients when considering whether a surgical procedure can be performed safely outside of the HLCC unit.

In order to provide bedside surgery safely in an HLCC unit, prior planning and performing a gap analysis to address the preoperative, intraoperative and postoperative phases is essential. All perioperative phases of care will be provided in the HLCC unit patient care room. Operating room (OR) staff should be involved in the development of all perioperative procedures and planning activities. All facility protocols should be followed with enhancements to maintain staff safety within the HLCC unit. There are many considerations to address for all phases of care when planning for surgical intervention in an HLCC unit.

Preoperative considerations to be addressed when developing surgical procedures include determining what equipment will be required, such as an operating table, back table, patient monitoring equipment, and procedural supplies. Ensure that the room possesses the required facility requirements, such as sufficient lighting, medical gases, and suction capabilities. Remove unnecessary equipment or furnishings from the room as well as covering necessary equipment with clear plastic covers to minimize exposure to the pathogen.

Intraoperative considerations include developing processes that maintain a sterile field, such as how to pass supplies into the room if needed. Attention should be given to utilizing methods that minimize the number of instruments required and include disposable instruments where appropriate. In addition, safer practices to minimize blood loss, such as using cautery rather than a scalpel to make incisions, should be explored. If cautery is not an option, the risk of staff injury can be eliminated or minimized by utilizing rounded rather than pointed scalpels, using tools to pick up sharp instruments or needles, and avoiding hand-to-hand passing of sharps by having a neutral passing zone in which sharps are placed prior to being picked up by another person.

Postoperative considerations to be addressed include the removal, decontamination, and sterilization of surgical instruments and equipment; the removal of both liquid and solid waste; and environmental cleanup and decontamination. Staffing for all 3 phases should include experienced OR staff who have been trained in and are knowledgeable about HLCC procedures. When performing surgical procedures within the NBU, during the intra- and postoperative phases PAPR-level PPE will be worn. During the intraoperative phase, sterile gown and gloves should also be worn over the PAPR-level PPE.

Radiology. The inclusion of X-ray diagnostics to evaluate a patient using portable digital imaging equipment should be considered when providing HLCC. A risk assessment should be completed to evaluate the availability of equipment and properly trained staff when deciding whether to offer X-rays for diagnostics. Radiology technologists who are willing to participate in the care of the patient in the HLCC unit and receive appropriate training in PPE and infection prevention and control (IPC) practices should be selected for the team. The NBU uses a portable X-ray machine and backup battery charger to obtain radiological images. These pieces of equipment are transported into the HLCC unit and stored in a designated clean room inside the NBU once the unit is activated. This equipment then remains within the NBU for the duration of the activation. Once the patient is discharged, or there is no further anticipated use of the X-ray equipment, the same decontamination process is applied to the X-ray machine as with all other equipment in the NBU: manual disinfection using appropriate Environmental Protection Agency (EPA) registered disinfectants and ultraviolet germicidal irradiation (UVGI) treatment.

When establishing the ability to provide X-ray services in an HLCC unit, SOPs should follow established facility protocols for placing orders and contacting designated staff using the existing electronic health record. The designated radiology technologist should utilize the same PPE donning and doffing methods in the unit as the rest of the HLCC staff, including assistance as needed as well as the standard observer system. The portable X-ray machine should be draped in protective plastic covers prior to moving them into the patient care areas.

When the radiology technologist is ready to enter the patient's room, the nurse(s) stationed inside serve to assist by ensuring adherence to safe entry and exit procedures. To minimize the extent of contamination and potential exposures, the radiology technologist should not have direct patient contact. Instead, they will verbally direct the nursing staff to correctly place the digital detector behind the patient for imaging. The digital detector can be contained in a plastic pouch designed for use in the HLCC unit to limit contamination of the equipment. The radiology technologist is then responsible for positioning the X-ray tube and making the exposure. Once the exposure has been made and the image has been transmitted, the HLCC unit front desk staff contact the radiologist for a preliminary reading. Once receipt of the image is confirmed and a preliminary report has been given, the radiology technologist can exit the patient care areas. The portable X-ray machine undergoes gross decontamination on exiting the patient care area hot zone and prior to placing it in the designated equipment holding area.

It should also be noted that the staff inside of the patient's room do not necessarily need to wear a lead apron when performing these X-rays. In order to reduce the amount of equipment needing decontamination and reduce risk of exposure from scatter radiation, the staff should remain at least 6 feet from the patient during X-ray exposure. If this is not feasible in the patient care area, additional risk assessments should be conducted to determine the safest procedures for the care space. In the event the patient is pregnant, a risk-benefit assessment should be performed by a perinatologist prior to the procedure. A dosimeter stick should also be placed on the portable X-ray machine to track the dose of each exposure.

Recovery Care

Patients in the convalescent stage of their illness require continued care during the recovery process. Patients in this stage should be monitored closely for development of secondary complications of the disease, medication reactions, and health care–associated infections. Depending on the disease, patients may require viral load monitoring or monitoring of other laboratory parameters during recovery. Physical therapy and occupational therapy may be engaged via telemedicine to assist the patient in recovery of their functional status. Attempts should be made to engage the patient in their recovery process and facilitate return to functional capacity, as feasible. Patients can assist with planning their daily schedule, participate in games or other activities, exercise, choose diet preferences, and visit with friends, family, and clergy via video technology.

Discharge and Follow-up

Discharge planning will vary depending on the disease process. In the United States, the Centers for Disease Control and Prevention (CDC), along with state and local public health authorities, should be consulted for guidance regarding criteria for discharge of patients with HHCDs. Based on these recommendations, the patient should be counseled about any necessary lifestyle modifications, including when it is safe to resume sexual activity, because some HHCDs may persist in body fluids for prolonged periods of time, despite recovery. General discharge discussions, including necessary medications, signs and symptoms to monitor for, and the scheduling of follow-up care should also occur. Prior to discharge, the HLCC physician team should communicate with any physicians who will be involved in follow-up care of the patient in order to provide clinical information and answer questions. Discharge planning should always include a case manager, who can provide assistance with transportation and coordinate follow-up care.

Behavioral Health Support

Patients treated in HLCC units are at risk for psychological distress, including symptoms of anxiety and depression. These reactions are due, in part, to the nature of the infection control procedures themselves. Reduced sensory stimulation, loss of control, limitations in social contact, and few meaningful activities may all contribute to the negative psychological consequences of treatment on an HLCC unit. Although there are no controlled studies of interventions designed to mitigate psychological distress in patients treated on such units, the qualitative-phenomenological literature, in connection with clinical experience, suggests a variety of strategies regarding the physical environment, staff-patient interaction, and patient autonomy, as summarized below.

Patient rooms should have a clock, calendar, windows (ideally with exterior views as well as onto the unit), artwork (such as nature scenes), games, reading material, exercise equipment, and shelving for personal belongings, including pictures from home. A telephone, television, computer/tablet, and internet access are vital for maintaining a connection to the outside world. In addition, when not medically contraindicated, patients should be allowed to keep snacks in their rooms rather than depending on staff for all meals.

Staff members should display identifying information outside their PPE by, for example, writing names across their gowns. Staff photographs and short biographical sketches, on paper or the web, could also be provided. It is recommended that all staff be educated on the psychological risks of isolation and strategies to mitigate such risks, including encouraging patients to express concerns, asking clarifying questions, and conveying understanding and empathy. Clear, consistent communication about infection control precautions and the reasons for their implementation is also essential, as patients may have trouble processing such information due to psychological and physical stress. In addition, instructions on infection control practices, as well as possible psychological reactions and recommended coping techniques, should be provided in written, verbal, and video-based formats to accommodate different learning styles. Providing ample opportunity for patients to ask (and to repeat) questions is critical. Professional interpreters should be consulted when necessary.

To combat feelings of helplessness and loss of control, staff should encourage patients to express preferences regarding visitors, the daily schedule, meals, lights/blinds, clothing, religious practices, and recreational activities (a small budget to purchase preferred supplies and reading materials is recommended). Staff should also allow patients to plan some uninterrupted time. Maximizing contact with family (through a secure audiovisual connection if necessary), consistent with patient wishes, is also critical. Accordingly, the hospital might consider designating a gathering space for family adjacent to the HLCC unit.

A behavioral health provider should screen all patients for preexisting and new-onset mental health conditions. The behavioral health provider can use psychological first aid (PFA) to assist patients with problem-solving, accessing social supports, and coping with treatment in the HLCC unit. PFA is a technique designed to reduce the occurrence of posttraumatic stress disorder, delivered by behavioral health specialists or trained health providers, who offer acute assistance to those affected as part of an organized response effort. Patients with acute stress and adjustment disorders due to traumatic deployments and/or the symptoms of the infectious disease may require ongoing treatment, including referral for medication.

HLCC unit personnel may be dealing with their own stressors, such as fear of infection, ostracism of their children at schools, and avoidance behaviors by friends and family members due to fear of contagion. Therefore, a behavioral health provider should also support the HLCC care team by fostering wellness and resilience prior to, during, and after unit activation.

Among children and adolescents, the above strategies must be adapted to an appropriate developmental level, and should include queries enabling an assessment of their understanding of the treatment and correcting misconceptions (e.g., the isolation precautions are a punishment); limiting and discussing exposure to media coverage of the infection; introducing hands-on activities to facilitate processing of feelings (e.g., playing, drawing); creating daily routines, including time for schoolwork; providing age-appropriate toys/crafts and child-friendly decor; finding ways for children to participate in their own care; encouraging parents to convey confidence in the HLCC staff; and, perhaps most importantly, maximizing contact with family and ensuring that it is predictable.

Family members of HLCC patients are subject to a broad range of emotional and economic stressors. Strategies to reduce family stress are essential to providing holistic care. Strategies include providing regular updates, especially when family members are away from the hospital; sharing information about normal family reactions, including fear of developing the illness; reminding families to use available social supports; cautioning about use of social media when the HLCC activation is covered by the press; and suggesting concrete activities for young family members to help their loved one (e.g., drawing a picture to decorate the hospital room). Facilities can also consider designating or employing a concierge nurse to assist with transportation, lodging, meals, patient contact, spiritual/religious needs, and regular contact with the medical team.

CHAPTER 10

Viral Hemorrhagic Fevers

MARK G. KORTEPETER

Introduction

The term "viral hemorrhagic fever" refers to a clinical syndrome caused by four families of single-stranded RNA viruses: filoviruses (Ebola and Marburg), arenaviruses (with "Old World" Lassa as the main concern, as well as the "New World" South American viruses, Machupo, Junin, and others), bunyaviruses (hantaviruses, Crimean Congo hemorrhagic fever [CCHF] virus, and Rift Valley fever virus), and flaviviruses (yellow fever, dengue, and others). Although the diseases caused by these viruses are frequently considered as a group based on their ability to cause a severe and deadly syndrome, many aspects of the diseases differ, including their natural hosts, geographic locations, annual incidence, prominent clinical features, and case fatality rates. The most important aspect considered in this chapter is the risk of spread in the nosocomial environment, which is primarily a concern for the filoviruses, arenaviruses, and CCHF. Filoviruses and arenaviruses are also considered potential agents of bioterrorism, because they can replicate well in cell culture and are infectious by the aerosol route, as demonstrated in animal studies— properties that are considered necessary for large-scale production and deployment. The large outbreak of Ebola virus disease in West Africa from 2014 to 2016 provides an example of the potential of these diseases to devastate a population, whether or not due to intentional spread, especially for the diseases that are communicable person to person where medical infrastructure is suboptimal.

Background

Hemorrhagic fever viruses are zoonotic pathogens that occur in their geographic settings based on the presence of a host, usually a small rodent or bat. Human cases result from direct or indirect contact with the animal's excretions, secretions, or blood. For example, African fruit bats are the presumed hosts of Ebola and Marburg viruses, and each of the arenaviruses has a specific rodent (mouse or rat) reservoir. Human infection by hemorrhagic fever viruses occurs by one of four general mechanisms, although the specific risk factors leading to infection may differ, depending on the virus:

1. Inhaling or ingesting excretions or secretions from rodent hosts (urine, feces). This applies to the arenaviruses (Lassa, South American VHFs) and bunyaviruses (hantaviruses), predominantly.

2. The bite of an infected mosquito (flaviviruses [yellow fever virus, dengue virus] and bunyaviruses [Rift Valley fever virus]) or tick (flaviviruses [Kyasanur forest disease, Omsk hemorrhagic fever virus] and bunyaviruses [CCHF]).

3. Contact with human or animal blood, body fluids, or tissues. This can occur in the occupational (animal slaughter, laboratory), hospital (filoviruses, arenaviruses, CCHF), or household setting.

4. Exposure to artificially generated aerosols in the context of a bioweapon attack or in the research laboratory setting (most VHFs, except dengue, which is not spread by aerosol, and CCHF viruses, which are difficult to grow in large quantities).

Contact with the virus usually occurs through a break in the skin, contact with mucous membranes, the respiratory tract, or occasionally through ingestion (e.g., consumption of bush meat for Ebola, or multimammate rats for Lassa). The primary means of infection during out-breaks has been through direct person-to-person contact, either in the health care or home environment. Significant spread has also occurred during burial rites where mourners have direct contact with the deceased and has also occurred from reuse of needles/syringes in locations with limited medical resources.

The incubation period for VHFs is generally 1–2 weeks following exposure. For the filoviruses, it is usually considered to be between 2 and 21 days, although most will become ill between the end of the first week and the middle of the second week. Individuals are generally not considered contagious until after the onset of symptoms and become more contagious as signs and symptoms worsen, and viral shedding in body fluids increases. Once ill, an individual should be considered contagious until full recovery and demonstration of an inability to detect virus by PCR. Individuals with filovirus infection may have prolonged shedding (for as long as 2 years) of virus in semen. Viral shedding in other VHF infections is less well characterized, and new information for Ebola is currently being developed through studies of Ebola survivors. The corpses of infected individuals should also be considered hazardous and buried in a manner that minimizes direct contact with the dead body.

Initial replication of Ebola virus occurs in monocytes and macrophages, followed by transport through the blood and lymphatics to target organs. These include the liver and spleen, although high concentrations of virus can be found in all major organs, including the heart and brain. The virus leads to necrosis and lymphocyte depletion as well as impairment of the endothelium and breakdown in the gastrointestinal mucosa.

Clinical illness generally begins with the acute onset of fever, malaise, prostration, skin flushing, conjunctival injection, myalgias, and occasionally sore throat (especially for Marburg and Lassa viruses). The viruses vary significantly in the prominence of other clinical features and severity of illness progression that they cause, but severe illness with any of them can be fatal. After the initial few days, patients infected with the filoviruses may develop significant loss of fluids from vomiting and diarrhea. Dengue fever, the filovirus infections, and Lassa fever frequently present with a maculopapular rash in the first week. Obtundation and encephalopathy occur with the filoviruses and New World arenaviruses.

All of the VHFs produce elevations in transaminases, but jaundice and icterus tend to occur more frequently with yellow fever and Rift Valley fever. Third-spacing of fluids leading to significant edema is most prominent with severe Lassa, but can occur with the filoviruses and hantaviruses, especially with the New World hantaviruses, where pulmonary edema is a prominent feature.

During the second week of illness, depending on several factors (viral virulence, route of exposure, inoculum, viremia level, host factors such as age), patients can progress to develop clotting abnormalities and thrombocytopenia that may manifest as oozing from venipuncture sites, petechiae, purpura, and ecchymoses. The viruses that typically lead to bleeding as a more prominent feature (Ebola, Marburg, CCHF, Lassa) are also the ones more frequently associated with nosocomial spread. Patients with severe disease may demonstrate a combination of neurologic and hematologic abnormalities. In rare cases, massive bleeding may occur, usually from the gastrointestinal tract.

Mortality rates for individual VHFs vary considerably. They can range from as high as 80–90% with the Ebola virus (historically referred to as the Zaire species of Ebola virus) or Marburg virus to less than 1% with Rift Valley fever. Among the five species of Ebola virus, the case fatality rates (CFRs) also vary widely, with the CFR for Ebola virus ranging between ~39 and 89%, Sudan virus averaging 53%, Bundibugyo virus 32%, Cote d'Ivoire virus 0% (only a single case), and Reston virus 0%. Reston virus has thus far failed to demonstrated human pathogenicity, despite individual animal handlers having seroconverted.

Despite the syndrome name of viral *hemorrhagic* fever, a minority of infected individuals will develop frank hemorrhage, and the majority who die do not succumb to blood loss alone. Instead, a sepsis-like clinical syndrome ensues in the more severe cases, with features including loss of vascular hemostasis and increased vascular permeability, decline in mean arterial pressure, lactic acidosis, shock, end organ failure, and death.

Diagnosis

The diagnosis of VHF should be considered in patients with an appropriate exposure history and a clinically compatible illness, such as fever with rash, transaminase elevation, and thrombocytopenia. Some cases, including those due to Lassa and the hantaviruses, as well as those with dengue hemorrhagic shock syndrome, may experience significant vascular leakage, causing hemoconcentration rather than anemia. VHFs, in their early stages, may mimic common diseases, which should be considered in the differential diagnosis in patients who have appropriate travel or other exposure histories. These common diseases include meningococcemia, other causes of bacterial sepsis, rickettsial infections, typhoid, and falciparum malaria. Usually a screening test for VHFs is done with RT-PCR, obtainable through the local or state health department laboratory, with confirmation done by the CDC. Other options for diagnosis, usually only available through containment laboratories, include viral culture, acute and convalescent serology, or immunohistochemistry on autopsy or other tissue specimens, which may need to be done in the absence of licensed tests for many of the pathogens. Patient specimens should be considered extremely hazardous and are best handled in BSL-3 or BSL-4 laboratories, when feasible, depending on the specific pathogen.

Treatment

There are no licensed therapies for any VHF; therefore, the primary aspect of care has been supportive: monitoring fluid status closely, monitoring and repleting electrolytes and glucose, minimizing procedures that may cause bleeding, and avoiding medications (such as NSAIDs) that may impair platelet function, use of blood products to correct deficits in hematocrit or other hematologic factors, vasopressors for hypotension, dialysis for renal failure, and ventilators for respiratory failure. The original Marburg outbreaks (in Marburg and Frankfurt, Germany, as well as the former Yugoslavia) in 1967 had a case fatality rate of 23%, which provided an early indicator that care in a developed setting might improve the case fatality rate when subsequent large outbreaks in Angola and the Democratic Republic of the Congo (DRC) led to mortality rates upwards of 80%. Close monitoring and judicious repletion of fluids has led to a significant decline in mortality from dengue hemorrhagic fever/shock syndrome. Using aggressive supportive care measures in developed-setting intensive care units in the United States and Europe led to lower case fatality rates (18.5%) than those that occurred in African Ebola treatment units, although the individuals cared for in the United States and Europe also received multiple investigational treatments, which may or may not have made a difference. In less developed settings, without ventilator support and renal dialysis, care must be taken to avoid overhydration and the risk of pulmonary edema. Significant strides have been made to bring the standard of care for VHF patients in field environments closer to that provided in developed settings, but there remain challenges in doing so.

Intravenous ribavirin has been used as an experimental treatment for several VHFs, including Lassa hemorrhagic fever, Argentine hemorrhagic fever, CCHF infection, and hemorrhagic fever renal syndrome (caused by Old World hantaviruses). Convalescent antibodies have also been used therapeutically against the arenaviruses, Lassa, and filoviruses, with varying effects.

Several different types of countermeasures are being assessed for use against the filoviruses, including immunotherapeutics (monoclonal and polyclonal antibody preparations), phsophorodiamidate morpholino oligomers (PMOs), lipid-encapsulated small interfering RNAs, small molecule inhibitors, and antiviral nucleoside analogs. Although some appear promising, few have been tested in robust clinical trials. Multiple products were tested, usually against historical controls in the large 2014–16 West Africa Ebola outbreak or given as emergency use investigational new drugs (INDs) in the United States and Europe. No conclusion can be made regarding safety or efficacy with those measures. Use of a cocktail of three monoclonal antibodies, ZMapp™, directed against the glycoprotein on the surface of Ebola Zaire appeared to reduce the case fatality rate in a randomized controlled trial, but the trial did not have adequate numbers to demonstrate statistical significance. In two 2018 outbreaks in the Democratic Republic of the Congo (DRC), several investigational products were approved for compassionate use: ZMapp™, two other monoclonal antibodies (single monoclonal Mab114 and triple monoclonal REGN3470-3471-3479), and the antiviral, remdesivir. As of this writing, a four-arm randomized controlled trial utilizing these products, with ZMapp™ serving as the control arm, is under way at certain Ebola treatment units in the DRC.

Prevention

The only VHF with a vaccine licensed in the United States is yellow fever. Investigational vaccines for many of the other VHFs are at varying stages of development, several of which have been tested in humans. For example, there are investigational vaccines for Junin virus (the vaccine is licensed in Argentina) and Rift Valley fever virus that have been used routinely for laboratory workers and have demonstrated protection in animals. Several vaccines have been tested against Ebola virus, and subsequently in humans, including DNA vaccines and adenovirus platforms. One that uses the vesiculostomatitis virus as a vector platform for the Ebola glycoprotein appeared to demonstrate protection against infection when it was used in a ring fashion in exposed household members during the 2014–16 Ebola outbreak in West Africa. It has been offered to health care workers and potentially exposed individuals in two subsequent outbreaks in the DRC in 2018, with more than 133,000 recipients as of this writing in the North Kivu outbreak. It has also been used for postexposure prophylaxis for a laboratory exposure as well as health care exposures in the field, based on the ability to protect nonhuman primates as postexposure prophylaxis.

Several vaccines against Marburg virus are also in development that have demonstrated the ability to protect in a nonhuman primate model, including recombinant VSV-vectored vaccines, adenovirus, and chimpanzee adenovirus-vectored vaccines. Some of these are undergoing early human testing. Some other vaccine platforms, such as DNA vaccines and viruslike particles, are being assessed in both animals and humans.

Outbreaks of VHFs that spread in the nosocomial environment have occurred most commonly in less developed settings, such as Africa or Asia, where health care and public health systems may be less robust. CCHF is an exception, given its wide distribution in developed and underdeveloped settings, and its occasional spread prior to recognition.

In general, in underdeveloped settings, basic hospital infection control modalities may be lacking due to limited resources and a consequent inability to purchase gloves, gowns, and eye protection, in addition to lack of robust laboratory infrastructure to allow early diagnosis before significant risk of spread occurs. Reuse of unsterilized needles has also led to explosive outbreaks. Significant reductions of spread to health care providers and family members in these environments can be accomplished using basic measures, such as triage, barrier methods to reduce caregiver contact with infectious body fluids, and staff education. Ensuring that caregivers understand the mechanisms of spread and demonstrate proficiency in proper donning and doffing of PPE can significantly reduce risk of spread.

Quarantine

Among the VHFs, only yellow fever is on the list of internationally quarantinable diseases. Quarantine is usually enforced in countries that have a recent risk of yellow fever outbreaks. Individuals are frequently required to provide documentation showing prior yellow fever vaccination, especially when entering the country from another yellow fever endemic country. Individuals with a syndrome clinically compatible with yellow fever could be quarantined until yellow fever was ruled out, not because of concern over person-to-person spread of the disease but rather due to the possibility of starting an outbreak through mosquito spread from a patient with active viremia.

By presidential executive order in the United States, yellow fever and other viral hemorrhagic fevers, specifically Marburg, Ebola, and CCHF, are quarantinable. Because of concerns of importation of Ebola virus into nonendemic countries during the West Africa outbreaks, the CDC conducted airport screening at those airports that were known hubs for flights returning from West Africa. Individuals with potential exposures were monitored by health departments for a period of 21 days for clinical illness. In some cases, health care providers who had cared for patients in West Africa were quarantined on return to the United States. The US military made the administrative decision to quarantine military personnel for 21 days on return from work in West Africa, even though they did not interact with patients. This was done for administrative purposes and for monitoring for potential other infections (Lassa, malaria). In high-risk laboratory exposures, laboratory workers have also been quarantined or actively monitored for 21 days.

In situations involving high-risk exposures, in the household, health care or laboratory setting, it is reasonable to monitor individuals for 21 days. Generally, quarantine is not necessary, because potential spread of the infection does not occur until after the onset of clinical illness, as long as the potentially exposed individuals can be relied on to follow up. They can be educated on recognizing early signs and symptoms, checking their temperature regularly, and maintaining regular contact with public health authorities. Whether or not a health care provider or laboratorian who has sustained a potential exposure is allowed to continue working during this period of time is a local institutional decision and would depend, in part, on the presumed risk of the exposure. Currently, there is no laboratory test that would identify reliably whether someone has been infected prior to the onset of illness. In fact, even after illness onset, current RT-PCR diagnostics may not become positive for 48–72 hours; therefore, repeating an initially negative test is reasonable 72 hours later, depending on the pretest probability that someone has been infected.

Individuals can be risk-stratified according to any potential exposure based on the following table:

High Risk—exposure to a patient with symptoms:

- Percutaneous or mucus membrane exposure to blood/body fluids
- Direct contact with a patient without PPE
- Processing lab specimens without PPE
- Direct contact with an infected dead body without PPE

Some Risk:

- Close contact with an infected individual in the household or health care/community setting without PPE
- Direct contact while wearing PPE
- Providing any direct patient care (not specifically for patients with a VHF) in a region of country with an active outbreak

Low Risk:

- Brief contact (shaking hands) with a patient in early stages without PPE

- In brief proximity with a patient in early stages (e.g., in the same room)

- Lab processing while wearing appropriate PPE

- Traveling on a plane with an infected patient without any identified high- or moderate- ("some") risk exposures

The utmost caution must be taken when caring for individuals infected with VHFs that have demonstrated risk of infecting laboratory workers or health care providers (filoviruses, Lassa, South American arenaviruses, CCHF) due to the potential for spread in the nosocomial environment. Individuals with signs or symptoms consistent with a VHF, and a consistent travel/exposure history should be isolated immediately away from other patients and staff and managed as persons under investigation (PUIs). The management of the PUI is addressed in chapter 6 of this manual.

In summary, health care facilities should have practiced procedures for the triage and identification of potentially exposed or ill patients with VHFs. Moreover, they must become familiar with those VHFs requiring quarantine and isolation and develop procedures for the expeditious diagnosis and appropriate disposition of potential VHF patients.

CHAPTER 11

Respiratory Diseases Potentially Warranting Care

In a High-Level Containment Care Unit

SHAWN VASOO

BRENDA ANG

YEE-SIN LEO

This chapter reviews the management of respiratory diseases that are associated with outbreaks and have pandemic potential. Although patients with these illnesses may be managed in a high-level containment care (HLCC) unit, several factors may affect this decision, including available resources and the number of cases. A guiding principle is that suspect or confirmed cases should be isolated and ideally cared for in a negative-pressure room, with attention paid to infection control and appropriate use of personal protective equipment (PPE) to prevent nosocomial disease propagation.

Severe Acute Respiratory Syndrome

Causative Agent. Severe acute respiratory syndrome (SARS) is caused by the SARS-coronavirus (SARS-CoV) a single-stranded (+) RNA virus (lineage B coronavirus) that emerged in Foshan in Guangdong Province, China, in November 2002. SARS was recognized as a syndrome in February 2003, and the causative coronavirus was identified in late March

2003. Bats are believed to be the reservoir, with the virus crossing species barriers and transmitting to other mammals (e.g., civets). Initial human infection is thought to be related to exposure to live, caged animals in game markets in southern China.

Historical Outbreaks and Current Status. The 2002–3 Guangdong outbreak spread by international travel, with major outbreaks occurring in Hong Kong, Vietnam, Singapore, Taiwan, and Toronto. The pandemic resulted in more than 8,096 cases and 774 deaths in 33 countries on 5 continents. The global outbreak was declared contained by the World Health Organization (WHO) on July 5, 2003. The virus continued to cause sporadic infections in Guangdong, with the last cluster related to infection acquired in a research laboratory in Beijing, which ended in May 2004.

No further cases have been detected worldwide since.

Route of Transmission, Attack Rates, R_o, and Nosocomial Acquisition. Spread between humans is primarily by mucosal contact with infectious droplets or fomites; the risk is heightened during aerosol-generating procedures (intubation, noninvasive ventilation, bronchoscopy, and nebulization). Airborne spread via infectious air plumes and fecal-oral contact facilitated by faulty sewage systems have been hypothesized in a large community outbreak in Amoy Gardens in Hong Kong and on aircraft. "Super-spreading events" noted in the outbreak were likely due to multiple factors including delay in isolation and the degree of viral shedding.

SARS has a basic reproduction number (R_o) of 3, which means that an infected individual would, on average, spread the disease to 3 others, if infection control measures are not instituted. One study noted an attack rate of 10–60% among nursing staff prior to recognition of the outbreak, and another 6.2% attack rate in households. A disproportionate number of health care workers (HCWs) were infected in this outbreak (40% in Singapore, 43.6% in Hong Kong), with the majority infected before recognition of this disease or the availability of a diagnostic test. One study found asymptomatic seroconversion in 7.5% of exposed health care workers. In the same study, asymptomatic SARS (seroconversion without clinical illness) was determined to be ~13% overall, but these cases were not thought to contribute significantly to secondary spread.

Case Fatality Rate. SARS has an estimated overall case fatality rate (CFR) of 9.6%. The CFR increases with age and is estimated to be ~15% in those 45–64 years, and > 50% in those 65 or older.

Isolation Precautions. Patients should be cared for in a negative-pressure isolation room (with 6–12 air changes per hour, an independent air supply and exhausted outside or HEPA filtered before recirculation), with the doors closed. Care in an HLCC unit is reasonable, given the high attack and case fatality rates. If not available, a regular isolation/single room with its own bathroom is an alternative, followed by a designated ward to cohort cases if the numbers increase. The disease is unforgiving if allowed to spread, so there is a strict need to follow appropriate infection control measures. For SARS, airborne (including droplet) and contact transmission precautions are advocated.

Personal Protective Equipment and Monitoring of Health Care Workers and Exposed Persons. HCWs should don gloves, gowns, and respiratory protection. It is not as clear whether eye protection is needed to prevent transmission, but goggles or a face shield are routinely recommended when within 3 feet of a SARS patient. For respiratory protection, disposable particulate respirators (N-95 or higher) or a powered air-purifying respirator (PAPR) are recommended, the latter especially for aerosol-generating procedures. Temperature monitoring for staff (e.g., twice to thrice daily) is recommended for up to 10 days after caring for a potential/confirmed SARS patient to detect HCW infection early.

Quarantine. Quarantine may be considered for 10 days from the last known exposure, depending on local regulations, for exposed (but asymptomatic) persons. Any HCW with potential exposure who develops symptoms should be evaluated promptly in an appropriate location for respiratory protection for SARS.

Transport of Patients. Movement of patients out of their rooms should be minimized. If this becomes necessary, patients should don a surgical mask and a clean patient gown and perform hand hygiene prior to transport. Considerations for ground and air transport, including the use of portable isolation units, can be found in the references and are addressed in detail in chapter 18.

Definitions for Suspect Cases (PUIs). SARS-CoV may reemerge and should be suspected in cases or clusters of severe and otherwise unexplained respiratory infections (fever > 38°C, cough/dyspnea and chest X-ray infiltrates) with a history of travel to areas of likely reemergence, such as mainland China, Hong Kong, or Taiwan (or contact with an ill traveler from those areas), exposure to a potential animal host (including exposure to or consumption of wild/exotic game animals), or work in an at-risk occupation, such as HCWs or laboratorians involved in SARS-CoV research. Once SARS-CoV reemerges anywhere in the world, the index of suspicion should be heightened and SARS should be suspected in patients with compatible symptoms and potential epidemiologic exposure.

Key Points in Clinical Care:

- Incubation period: An incubation period averaging 6.4 days (range 2–10 days, maybe as long as 16 days).

- Clinical symptoms: An influenza-like illness, fever > 38°C (in most patients), lower respiratory tract symptoms (cough, dyspnea); a minority of cases may be present with mild or atypical presentations (e.g., diarrhea or lack of fever).

- Diagnosis: Laboratory testing is usually via RT-PCR, with an oro- or nasopharyngeal swab and a second specimen source, such as serum/plasma in the first week of illness, and stool after the first week of illness. Confirmation requires two positive specimens (from different sources or the same source, on different days). PCR may be falsely negative in respiratory samples especially early in the course of illness (before day 3–5) as viral shedding increases and peaks only around day 11. Paired serology using immunofluorescent antibody (IFA) or enzyme-linked immunosorbent assay (ELISA) may also be helpful. These are positive usually only after the end of the second week of illness. Lymphopenia and a raised lactate dehydrogenase level are also common among SARS patients, the latter portending a poor prognosis.

- Treatment: Treatment is supportive. Ribavirin, steroids, and lopinavir/ritonavir, interferon (type I), intravenous immunoglobulin, and convalescent sera have been utilized, but efficacy is unknown and some treatments may even cause harm (e.g., secondary infections with steroids). No vaccine is available. Extracorporeal membrane oxygenation (ECMO) may be helpful in acute respiratory distress syndrome (ARDS), extrapolating from the experiences with H7N9 influenza and Middle Eastern respiratory syndrome (MERS).

- Period of infectivity: Patients should be considered infectious until 10 days after resolution of symptoms (e.g., fever and respiratory). Dried virus in the environment may be infective for an estimated 6 days.

- Management of patient waste: Medical waste has not been associated with spread of disease; therefore, SARS-CoV contaminated medical waste is handled as per facility-specific/state/local procedures for routine medical (biohazardous) waste.

- Cautions: Avoid cough-inducing procedures and use of noninvasive positive pressure ventilation (e.g., BiPAP), as these may lead to aerosolization of infectious particles. A hydrophobic submicron viral/bacterial filter should be placed between the endotracheal tube and the ventilator circuit tubing and a second filter in the expiratory limb of the ventilator to minimize risk of aerosolization.

Middle East Respiratory Syndrome

Causative Agent. MERS was first recognized in June 2012 in a Saudi patient with acute respiratory distress syndrome (ARDS) and renal failure who expired 11 days after admission. The causative agent, the novel MERS-coronavirus (CoV; the first lineage C coronavirus known to infect humans), was identified in September 2012. The earliest human cases were identified retrospectively in a Jordanian nosocomial outbreak in April 2012. Dromedary camels are the reservoir, and zoonotic transmission is thought to be primarily due to close animal-human contact (e.g., contact with respiratory secretions or consumption of raw camel milk, urine, or meat).

Historical Outbreaks and Current Status. Since its emergence (and as of the end of July 2018), there have been a total of 2,237 laboratory-confirmed cases of MERS in 27 countries worldwide with 793 deaths (CFR 35.5%), with 80% reported from Saudi Arabia. Travel-related cases have occurred outside the Middle East, with a large and notable outbreak in South Korea in May–July 2015, in which 186 confirmed infections arose from an ill returned traveler from Saudi Arabia. Cases continue to be reported in the Arabian Peninsula.

Route of Transmission, Attack Rates and R_o and Nosocomial Acquisition. Although MERS-CoV has an estimated overall R_o of < 1 and appears to be less transmissible than SARS-CoV, infections have occurred in the young and healthy, and it has a predilection for the immunocompromised, including diabetics and persons with renal failure and chronic lung disease, leading to a higher overall CFR. MERS-CoV transmission is thought to occur primarily via droplets, but transmission by fomites and aerosols may also occur. Amplification in health care settings has been a significant issue, with attack rates (seroconversion) found to range between 2.4% (physicians) and 29.4% (radiology technicians) in one Saudi hospital. Since July 21, 2018, 38% (17 of 45) of secondary cases reported to the WHO were health care–associated (occurring in HCWs, other exposed patients, family visitors); 66% (37 of 56) of community-acquired MERS cases were associated with dromedary contact (direct or indirect).

Case Fatality Rate. MERS has a crude CFR of 35.5%, and risk of mortality is higher in older males with underlying medical conditions (e.g., diabetes, renal failure, and hypertension).

Isolation Precautions. As with SARS, patients should be cared for with the doors closed in a negative-pressure isolation room (with 6–12 air changes per hour, an independent air supply and exhausted outside or HEPA filtered before recirculation), and precautions should be taken for airborne (including droplet) and contact transmission. Care in an HLCC unit, if feasible, is a reasonable consideration.

Personal Protective Equipment and Monitoring of Health Care Workers and Exposed Persons. HCWs should don gloves, gowns, and respiratory and eye protection. For respiratory protection an N-95 disposable particulate respirator or a PAPR is recommended, especially for aerosol-generating procedures. Temperature monitoring for staff (e.g., twice daily) has also been used to detect HCW infection, and such monitoring should continue for up to 14 days after caring for a potential/confirmed MERS patient, regardless of the individual's use of PPE. Staff with unprotected exposures to MERS patients may need to be placed under controlled monitoring for development of illness or potential exclusion from work for 14 days.

Transport of Patients. Avoid movement of patients out of their isolation rooms as much as feasible. As with SARS, if this becomes necessary, patients should don a surgical mask and clean gown, and perform hand hygiene before movement out of rooms. Guidance regarding air transport may be found in the references, while ground transport recommendation follows that for SARS.

Definitions for Suspect Cases (PUIs). MERS should be suspected in persons with severe illness (fever and pneumonia/ARDS) who have traveled (or who are contacts of an ill traveler with a respiratory illness) to the Arabian Peninsula within 14 days of symptom onset, or who are part of a suspect MERS cluster. MERS should also be suspected in persons with milder illness (e.g., fever or respiratory symptoms) with exposure to a health care facility in the Arabian Peninsula where there has been recent MERS transmission or who are contacts of a known MERS case, within 14 days of symptom onset.

Key Points in Clinical Care:

- Incubation period: 2–14 days (median 5–6 days), however, in rare cases (e.g., immunocompromised) may extend to as long as 21 days.
- Clinical symptoms: Mild cases—Low grade fever, rhinorrhea, sore throat, myalgias, influenza-like illness. Severe cases–dyspnea, ARDS.
- Diagnosis: Multiple specimens (whenever possible, *both* upper AND lower respiratory specimens, ideally within 7 days of onset of illness) should be obtained for PCR-based testing. As ~21% of cases may be mild or asymptomatic, WHO recommends testing of all close contacts of MERS patients (including HCWs). Lower respiratory specimens (e.g., bronchoalveolar lavage, sputum, and tracheal aspirates) contain the highest viral loads. Upper

respiratory specimens (e.g. naso- or oropharyngeal swabs) may also detect the virus, but every attempt should be made to test lower tract specimens in patients strongly suspected for MERS and/or who have lower tract disease. A single negative test does not satisfactorily rule out disease, and repeat testing is recommended. Serologic testing (e.g., IFA, ELISA, with confirmation via a neutralization assay) may also be useful (single sample if > 14 days have elapsed since illness onset, or paired samples 3–4 weeks apart) in diagnosing cases and for detecting asymptomatic transmissions, although cross-reactions with other coronaviruses may be problematic. The CDC suggests serum for RT-PCR testing in the first 10–12 days of illness; however, lower levels of viremia may make serum/plasma less useful as a diagnostic specimen for MERS as compared to SARS. Limited data from 21 patients presenting with a median of 2 days (range 0–12 days) from symptom onset to diagnosis in the 2015 Korean outbreak found viremia in only 7 (33%) of patients, but this was associated with a worse outcome, including mortality.

- Treatment: Treatment is supportive, and patients with ARDS may benefit from ECMO, which may lower mortality. The efficacy of ribavirin, steroids, lopinavir/ritonavir, interferon, and intravenous immunoglobulin are uncertain and should not be used outside of a clinical trial. Convalescent sera may be helpful, but robust clinical data are lacking and titers in recovered individuals may not be sufficiently high. Several early vaccine and immunotherapy trials are under way.

- Period of infectivity: The duration of infectivity is unclear. It is currently recommended that patients be placed on transmission-based precautions for at least 24 hours beyond the resolution of clinical illness, with two respiratory specimens (preferably lower respiratory tract) negative for MERS-CoV by PCR collected 24 hours apart.

- Management of patient waste: MERS-CoV–contaminated medical waste is handled as per facility-specific/state/local procedures for routine medical (biohazardous) waste.

- Cautions: Avoid cough-inducing procedures and use of noninvasive positive pressure ventilation (e.g., BiPAP) as these may lead to aerosolization of respiratory secretions. A hydrophobic submicron viral/bacterial filter should be placed between the endotracheal tube and the ventilator circuit tubing and a second filter in the expiratory limb of the ventilator to reduce the risk of aerosolization.

Novel/Avian Influenza

Causative Agent. Influenza is caused by a single-stranded (−) RNA virus, and novel lineages, mostly of avian or swine origin, emerge periodically due to genetic reassortment. These have caused human disease, including pandemics (e.g., the 2009 H1N1 virus). H5, H7, H9, and H10 avian subtypes are primarily zoonoses with limited transmission to humans. H5N1 and H7N9, which have caused severe disease and, to date, limited outbreaks in humans, will be the focus of this section. Concerns remain regarding the possibility that novel influenza strains might further adapt to humans, causing another pandemic.

Historical Outbreaks and Current Status. H5N1 emerged in Hong Kong in 1997 and reemerged in mainland China in 2003, while H7N9 emerged in 2013 in China. Both viruses have spilled over from birds and caused human infections, but person-to-person spread is currently limited and non-sustained. H5N1 is a highly pathogenic avian influenza (HPAI) causing severe disease in poultry and has spread geographically due to migratory birds, while H7N9 has emerged as a lowly pathogenic avian influenza (LPAI) causing little or no symptoms in poultry, but HPAI variants emerged in November 2016, and these have also caused human infections. As of July 2018, WHO has reported 860 cases of H5N1 in 16 countries, with 454 deaths (52.8% mortality).

Since February 2013, H7N9 has caused annual winter outbreaks in China. As of March 2018, there have been 1,567 H7N9 laboratory-confirmed cases with 615 (39.2%) deaths. Most H7N9 cases have occurred in mainland China with the worst wave thus far in 2016–17, and the few cases (numbers in parentheses) from other territories/countries were linked to travel to mainland China: Hong Kong (21), Macao (2), Taiwan (6), Malaysia (1), and Canada (2).

Route of Transmission, Attack Rates and R_o, and Nosocomial Acquisition. Human infection with avian influenza is primarily via exposure with infected birds (live or dead); about 60–75% of human H5N1 and H7N9 infection report recent exposure. Potential routes of infection include inhalation of infectious droplets, airborne droplet nuclei, and possibly self-contamination of facial mucous membranes following fomite contact, or ingestion. Person-to-person transmission is thought to be rare and is not sustained, occurring only when there is prolonged and close contact. The estimated R_o is 1.14 for H5N1 and between 0.1 and 0.47 for H7N9. The household attack rate for H5N1 was estimated to be 18.3% and secondary attack rate to be 3.1–4.5% in an Indonesian study. The secondary attack rate of H7N9 has been estimated to be ~1.3–2.2%. HCW acquisition of H5N1 has been reported in a Vietnamese nurse who developed clinical illness, and asymptomatic seroconversion to H5N1 has been found in 4% of exposed HCWs in Hong Kong, but this appears to be low as several studies have found a lack of clinical illness or seroconversion in exposed HCWs. Small clusters of patient-to-patient and probable patient-to-HCW nosocomial spread of H7N9 have been described, but as in the case of H5N1, no sustained transmission has been observed.

Case Fatality Rate. It is not entirely clear why H5N1 has an overall higher CFR of 52.8% (to date, as of July 2018), compared to H7N9 (39.2%, as of March 2018), despite the latter's predilection for older individuals.

Isolation Precautions. Similar to patients with SARS and MERS, patients should be cared for in a negative-pressure isolation room with the doors closed (with 6–12 air changes per hour, an independent air supply and exhausted outside or HEPA filtered before recirculation), and precautions should be taken against airborne (including droplet) and contact transmission. Cohorting may be considered when there are large numbers of infected patients requiring isolation.

Personal Protective Equipment and Monitoring of Health Care Workers and Exposed Persons. Health care workers should don gloves, gowns, and respiratory and eye protection. For respiratory protection an N-95 disposable particulate respirator or a PAPR is recommended, especially during aerosol-generating procedures. Staff caring for patients with suspected/confirmed novel influenza should be monitored for illness. Analogous to SARS/MERS, temperature monitoring for staff (e.g., twice daily) may be considered to detect HCW infection. Symptom monitoring should continue for up to 10 days after caring for a potential/confirmed novel influenza patient. Staff/persons with unprotected exposures to novel influenza patients should be excluded from work for 10 days and be monitored for development of illness. Extended monitoring for a further 10 days (i.e., 20 days total) was used in a Hong Kong unit for 70 HCWs with unprotected exposures to H7N9, but no HCW infections were noted.

Transport of Patients. Avoid movement of patients out of their isolation rooms if possible. If movement becomes necessary, patients should don a surgical mask and clean gown, and should perform hand hygiene before movement out of rooms. Avoid aerosol-generating procedures during ground transportation, and disinfect the cabin of the ambulance and equipment with phenolics, bleach, or quaternary ammonium compounds after the patient is transferred out. No specific guidance for air or ground transport is available from the CDC for avian influenza, although the guidelines for MERS/SARS are available as references.

Definitions for Suspect Cases (PUIs). Novel/avian influenza should be suspected in persons with an influenza-like illness, and in particular, patients with clinical or radiologic evidence of pneumonia or a severe, unexplained respiratory illness who have had a potential exposure within the preceding 10 days, such as close contact with a confirmed or suspect case of avian influenza, travel to at-risk areas where avian influenza is circulating, exposure to infected birds/animals, or work in a laboratory that handles novel/avian influenza.

Key Points in Clinical Care:

- Incubation period: H7N9 influenza, median 6 (range, 1–10 days), H5N1 influenza, median 4 (range 2–8 days).

- Clinical symptoms: An influenza-like illness (fever, with cough or sore throat). Fever ($\geq$ 38°C) and cough are the most common symptoms but are less common in H5N1 (65% and 54%, respectively) compared to H7N9 (79% and 71%, respectively). Sore throat seems to be uncommon for both H5N1/H7N9 influenza (5–9%). Severe cases—pneumonia, dyspnea, ARDS.

- Diagnosis: Obtain respiratory specimens (nasopharyngeal swab or nasal aspirate/wash, or oropharyngeal swab; lower respiratory tract specimens are preferred if there is pneumonia, e.g., bronchoalveolar lavage or endotracheal tube aspirate) as soon as possible after the onset of illness (before day 7 of illness if possible) for testing via PCR. It is prudent to obtain multiple specimens from different sites on at least two consecutive days. Commercial assays may yield an "influenza A, unsubtypeable" result or may fail to detect novel influenza due to lower analytic sensitivity. Patients with suspected novel/avian influenza or unsubtypeable influenza A results should have further testing performed at state or public health laboratories (e.g., the CDC or a WHO collaborating center).

- Treatment: The neuraminidase inhibitors (NAIs) are the mainstay of pharmacotherapy for patients with novel influenza, and antiviral treatment should be started as soon as possible regardless of time elapsed from illness onset (but ideally within 48 hours) for all confirmed and probable cases, as clinical benefit may still be derived. Treatment should not be delayed because of pending laboratory results, and may be extended (e.g., 10 days or longer) in severely ill or immunocompromised patients who may shed virus for longer periods and who are at risk of developing resistant virus.

- Chemoprophylaxis: Both the CDC and WHO recommend antiviral chemoprophylaxis at *treatment doses* (e.g., with oseltamivir 75 mg BID for 5 days if renal function is normal), rather than the usual seasonal influenza prophylaxis doses (e.g., oseltamivir 75 mg daily for 10 days) for close contacts based on the assumption that infection may have already occurred and given the concerns of emergence of antiviral resistance in cases of prophylaxis failure as seen in the 2009 H1N1 pandemic. Close contact is defined as unprotected exposure within 6 feet/2 meters of an infected person for a prolonged time or contact with infectious secretions 1 day before onset of clinical illness till resolution of illness. Chemoprophylaxis may be extended (e.g., to 10 days) if exposure is likely to be ongoing (e.g., due to potential prolonged shedding of virus in undiagnosed contacts).

- Other treatments: Convalescent plasma or hyperimmune immunoglobulin may be helpful. Corticosteroids have increased the risk of secondary bacterial infection and mortality, and their use cannot be recommended routinely. Other immunomodulatory treatments such as statins, sirolimus, and macrolides have been utilized, but there is currently no clear evidence of benefit versus harm. Patients with ARDS may benefit from ECMO, which may lower mortality.

- Antiviral resistance: H5N1 and H7N9 are generally susceptible to NAIs. Although uncommon, resistance may occur; for example, in H7N9 the R292K mutation confers resistance to oseltamivir and peramivir, with decreased susceptibility to zanamivir. The H275Y mutation confers high-level resistance to oseltamivir, and reduced susceptibility to peramivir in H5N1 viruses (zanamivir retains susceptibility). Some H5N1 strains may be susceptible to the M2 inhibitors (amantadine and rimantadine), although most H7N9 strains are not. The NAI laninamavir (administered by inhalation, approved in Japan) shows a similar profile to zanamivir and is undergoing phase III trials. Favipiravir, a viral RNA-dependent RNA polymerase inhibitor, has activity against NAI-resistant strains and broad activity against RNA viruses and has been approved for stockpiling in Japan. The role of the new viral PA subunit polymerase inhibitor baloxavir (FDA-approved in 2018) remains to be defined but holds promise given its novel mechanism of action, rapid virological effect, single-dose strategy, and potential for synergy with NAIs, but emerging resistance remains a concern.

- Vaccines: Not widely available, but some countries, including the United States, stockpile H5N1 and H7N9 vaccines. These may be considered for first responders to human/animal outbreaks or in designated referral facilities for novel influenza, but it is uncertain whether these vaccines would be adequately immunogenic matches to an eventual outbreak strain caused by an ever-evolving virus.

- Period of infectivity: For seasonal influenza, patients are considered infectious for 7 days from the onset of illness or at least 24 hours after resolution of fever and respiratory symptoms, whichever is longer. Less information is available for avian influenza; however, recent data from patients with H7N9 indicate a median duration of RNA detection from respiratory specimens of 15.5 days, and this could extend up to 30 days in those who are immunocompromised, receive corticosteroids, had a delay in NAI treatment, and had a fatal course. H5N1 RNA has also been detectable for up to 27 days in the lower respiratory tract in patients with fatal disease. No specific recommendations are available for novel influenza, but given these data, patients with novel influenza should be placed on isolation precautions for ≥ 24 hours after resolution of clinical illness (or ≥ 7 days from onset of illness, whichever is longer), and units may consider testing (e.g., evaluation by PCR for two negative respiratory samples 24 hours apart as for MERS-CoV) prior to removing from isolation.

- Management of patient waste: Medical waste from patients with novel influenza is handled as per facility-specific/state/local procedures for routine medical (biohazardous) waste.

- Cautions: Avoid cough-inducing procedures and use of noninvasive positive pressure ventilation (e.g., BiPAP) as these may lead to aerosolization of secretions. A hydrophobic submicron viral/bacterial filter should be placed between the endotracheal tube and the ventilator circuit tubing and a second filter in the expiratory limb of the ventilator to reduce risk of aerosolization.

CHAPTER 12

Orthopoxviruses

GEORGE F. RISI

Variola Virus (Smallpox)

HISTORY

Smallpox has been one of humankind's greatest scourges since before recorded history. Few diseases, including plague, yellow fever, or cholera have impacted human populations and history as dramatically. The origin of smallpox is obscure, but it is believed to have appeared at the time of the first agricultural settlements in northeastern Africa around 10,000 BCE. The original animal reservoir was probably a rodent that has since become extinct. In small populations, the disease would burn itself out once all members of the village or community had been infected, and not until population densities of about 200,000 developed was it able to sustain itself in humans. The earliest evidence of skin lesions resembling those of smallpox is found on the faces of mummies from the time of the 18th and 20th Egyptian dynasties (1570 to 1085 BCE) and on the well-preserved mummy of Ramses V, who died as a young man in 1157 BCE. The first recorded smallpox epidemic occurred in 1350 BCE during the Egyptian-Hittite wars. The illness was passed to the Hittite population by Egyptians, infecting the Hittite king, Suppiluliumas I, and his heir, Arnuwandas, and precipitating a sharp decline in their civilization.

Smallpox greatly affected the development of Western civilization. Smallpox and measles were introduced into the New World by the Spanish, and over the course of about 100 years between 1518 and 1620, the population of Mexico declined from 25 million to 1.6 million, in part due to such infection introductions. In Europe, by the end of the 18th century, an estimated 400,000 persons died annually from smallpox, and survivors accounted for one-third of all cases of blindness. During the 18th century, 5 reigning European monarchs died of smallpox, and the Austrian Hapsburg line of succession shifted 4 times in 4 generations.

MICROBIOLOGY

Smallpox is caused by variola (from Latin the diminutive *varius,* meaning spotted) virus, a DNA virus member of the genus *Orthopoxvirus* in the *Poxviridae* family. The orthopoxviruses are among the largest and most complex of all viruses, which serologically cross-react, and appear to offer cross-protection against infection. Smallpox is caused by two closely related but genetically distinct viruses, *Variola major* (typical smallpox) and *Variola minor* (alastrim). Clinically they are similar, but *Variola minor* cases are associated with fewer symptoms, less extensive rash, less scarring, and much lower mortality. Three other members of the *Orthopoxvirus* family also cause disease in humans: vaccinia (the basis of current smallpox vaccines), monkeypox (see below), and cowpox.

PATHOGENESIS OF DISEASE

The infectious dose for variola is unknown but may be as low as only a few virions. Typical infection begins after deposition of the virus on the oropharyngeal or respiratory mucosa. The virus is usually transmitted by contact or in droplets expressed from nasal and oropharyngeal secretions. While cough is not a typical symptom of smallpox, when cough is present the virus can be expelled as a fine-particle aerosol. After replication in local tissues, the virus then migrates to, and multiplies in, regional lymph nodes.

Asymptomatic viremia develops on about the 3rd or 4th day, with virus migrating from regional nodes to the organs of the reticuloendothelial system including liver, spleen, bone marrow, and distant lymph nodes, where replication continues. Secondary viremia begins on about the 8th day and is followed by clinical manifestations. The virus, contained in leukocytes, then localizes in small blood vessels of the dermis and below the oral and pharyngeal mucosa, where it subsequently infects adjacent cells, leading to the typical manifestations of exanthem and enanthem.

CLINICAL MANIFESTATIONS

The incubation period is characteristically 12 days, with a range of 7–17. The first clinical sign of infection is a prodromal illness, corresponding with the secondary viremia phase, characterized by the abrupt onset of malaise, fever that may exceed 40°C, constitutional symptoms, vomiting, and delirium. Around the 3rd or 4th day buccal and pharyngeal lesions begin to appear. Rash begins on the face and spreads to the forearms and hands, and then to the lower limbs and trunk. Lesions, which are always more prominent on the face, begin as macules and quickly evolve to papules and then to vesicles over a few days. Pustules appear about the 8th day of illness. The round and tense pustules are deeply embedded in the dermis and thus are firm to the touch. Pustules eventually dry and form scabs, which leave scars after flaking off.

Mortality from *Variola major* was reported to be from 20% in some communities to as high as > 50% in totally naive communities such as Native Americans. The most commonly quoted overall mortality rate is 30%. However, since the virus was eliminated 4 decades ago before the onset of the HIV pandemic and medical advances allowing longer survival of immunocompromised individuals of all types, and most individuals do not receive the vaccine, the untreated mortality rate today would be expected to be much higher. Death, if it occurred, usually happened in the second week of illness and was attributed to immune complex mediated shock. More severe clinical presentations believed to be related to impaired cellular immune response yielded hemorrhagic or "flat type" smallpox cases, who never developed the typical smallpox lesions; these infections were nearly universally fatal.

DIFFERENTIAL DIAGNOSIS

Clinical diagnosis remains the most important step for suspecting and ultimately confirming a reemergence of smallpox. Febrile exanthems are common, and many eruptive skin lesions were historically misinter-preted as smallpox. Severe varicella (chicken pox) and monkeypox are probably the diseases most likely to be misidentified, as well as erythema multiforme with bullae, disseminated herpes zoster, impetigo, and severe contact dermatitis. On rare occasions, patients who are immunized with the smallpox vaccine (vaccinia) can develop disseminated vaccinia infection. A careful history and physical will be important in establishing the correct diagnosis. Typical smallpox always begins with a febrile prodrome prior to the exanthem. In addition, lesions are centrifugal in distribution (concentrated in the face and distal extremities, while more sparing on the trunk), and they progress in slow synchrony. With varicella, lesions are more centrally distributed, evolve rapidly and at different stages, and generally appear concurrently with onset of fever. Varicella lesions are delicate and superficial (dewdrops on a rose petal), and are almost never found on the palms or soles, as opposed to variola lesions, which are firm and deep. Monkeypox lesions are quite similar to small-pox, but monkeypox infections are often distinguishable by epidemiology and the frequent presence of cervical and inguinal lymphadenopathy.

DIAGNOSIS

The identification of even a single suspected case of smallpox should be treated as an international health emergency and brought immediately to the attention of national officials through local and state health departments.

The Centers for Disease Control and Prevention (CDC) has developed a diagnostic algorithm for clinicians (see https://www.cdc.gov/smallpox /clinicians/algorithm-protocol.html). Specimens for testing of potential smallpox patients should only be collected by an individual who has been recently vaccinated (or is vaccinated that day) and is wearing appropriate personal protective equipment (PPE). Vesicular or pustular fluid is obtained by opening the lesions with the blunt end of a scalpel. The fluid is then absorbed onto a cotton swab. Alternatively, scabs can be picked off with a forceps. Specimens should be bagged or stoppered and then placed in a sealed, puncture-proof container for transport. The CDC maintains a website where specifics and assistance can be provided (http://emergency.cdc.gov/agent/smallpox/response-plan/files/guide-d .pdf) and their hotline number is 800-232-4636 (800-CDCINFO).

Orthopox infection can be confirmed rapidly by electron microscopic (EM) examination of vesicular or pustular fluid or scabs. Although all orthopoxviruses exhibit identically appearing brick-shaped virions, the history and clinical picture should help differentiate the illness from cowpox, monkeypox, or vaccinia infections. Definitive laboratory identification and characterization of the virus involves growth of the virus in cell culture or on chorioallantoic egg membrane and characterization of strains by use of various biologic assays, including polymerase chain reaction, and restriction fragment length polymorphism.

TREATMENT

While some weak evidence suggested mortality reduction with use of vaccinia immune globulin (VIG) or convalescent serum, no universally accepted or licensed therapeutics existed for smallpox prior to eradication. Fortunately, renewed emphasis on smallpox countermeasures in US civilian and military biodefense research in the early 2000s resulted in a number of new candidates, including tecovirimat (TPOXX®, formerly ST-246), a new orthopoxvirus-specific antiviral drug. In July 2018, oral tecovirimat was approved in the United States for treatment of smallpox in adults and pediatric patients weighing ≥ 13 kg. The recommended dosage of tecovirimat for those weighing ≥ 40 kg is 600 mg BID. For pediatric patients weighing between 25 and 40 kg, the dose is 400 mg BID, and for those between 13 and 25 kg, 200 mg BID. The duration of treatment is 14 days. An intravenous formulation of the product is undergoing phase I development. This agent is only available through the US government's Strategic National Stockpile (SNS). Cidofovir, an FDA-licensed intravenous antiviral, has also been shown to have efficacy against orthopoxviruses in animal models of infection. Brincidofovir is an analog of cidofovir formulated for oral administration that may have fewer adverse effects compared to cidofovir. It is undergoing testing as an additional therapeutic agent.

VACCINES

All smallpox vaccines currently in use are derived from vaccinia virus, an orthopoxvirus whose origins and natural host are unknown. The most commonly used vaccine strain in the United States was the New York

City Board of Health strain from which Dryvax and then ACAM2000 were derived. Dryvax, the previous stockpiled standard US vaccinia vaccine, has been phased out, and the vaccine that is currently used is ACAM2000, derived from Dryvax but grown in cell culture. The SNS currently stockpiles sufficient ACAM 2000 to vaccinate the entire US population if needed. Other countries used different strains of vaccinia virus, including the Lister (or Elestree) strain (UK), EM-63 (Russia), Temple of Heaven (China), Padwadanger (India), and LC16m8 (Japan). While all appear to have relatively similar efficacy, the frequency of adverse events may vary by strain.

For individuals with a recent history of smallpox exposure, postexposure vaccination as soon as feasible and within up to 96 hours may prevent, or at least ameliorate, disease. While not approved for post exposure prophylaxis, tecovirimat offers an alternative to this, with minimal side effects. Use of tecovirimat as PEP would be a topic for discussion in the event of an outbreak of smallpox.

Vaccine is administered via scarification and results in development of an eschar (the only marker for successful vaccination), which leaves a visible scar in most individuals and therefore permanent evidence of vaccination. Vaccination is often associated with fever, local inflammation, and lymphadenopathy. Historically, the vaccine caused more severe side effects in approximately 75 per one million recipients. The most commonly reported serious adverse events are progressive vaccinia (vaccinia necrosum), eczema vaccinatum, and vaccinial encephalitis, and death occurs in roughly one per million primary vaccinees. Adverse events are most commonly seen after initial vaccination, and frequency diminishes dramatically with subsequent administrations. Contraindications to receipt of ACAM 2000 in the nonemergency setting include patients with immunodeficiencies, individuals with eczema or other exfoliative skin condition, pregnant women, anaphylaxis to polymyxin and neomycin (trace amounts of these agents are present in the vaccine), or close contacts with immunocompromised patients. In situations with bona fide exposures to smallpox, vaccination with a live vaccinia preparation has historically been considered reasonable despite typical contraindications, although modified vaccinia Ankara (MVA) might now be considered an alternative.

In 2003 the US Department of Health and Human Services implemented a smallpox vaccination program with Dryvax for potential first responders. In 38,000 administrations, there were 822 reported adverse events, 100 of which were considered serious. Adverse events included myocarditis and pericarditis (21 cases) and unexpected ischemic cardiac events (10 cases). On the basis of this, additional contraindications to the vaccine were added, of either a history of cardiac disease or the presence of 3 major risk factors for atherosclerotic heart disease (hypertension, diabetes, hypercholesterolemia, smoking, or a history of heart disease in a first-degree relative before the age of 50).

MVA, manufactured under the name Imvamune, is a third-generation nonreplicating vaccine that has been used in a number of human trials and is currently approved for use in Europe and Canada. It has an improved safety profile in humans when compared to replication competent smallpox vaccines, but its efficacy is not as well characterized. It is intended for use in individuals for whom the use of ACAM 2000 is contraindicated. The vaccine is administered as a 0.5 ml subcutaneous injection at days 0 and 28 for primary vaccines. There is no eschar associated with this product. Imvamune is an investigational product that is also stored in the SNS.

ISOLATION

Suspected smallpox patients should be placed under contact and airborne isolation. Patients are most infectious from the onset of the enanthem through the first 7–10 days of rash. The infectiousness of an individual patient is primarily related to the extent and severity of the enanthem in the mouth and throat. As scabs form, even though the scabs contain large amounts of viable virus, the virions appear to be tightly bound to the fibrin matrix and thus pose much less risk of transmission. Despite that, patients should be considered potentially contagious until all eschars have fallen off.

Transmission of smallpox generally occurred with prolonged and extensive contact, and secondary cases were most commonly seen in those who lived with or cared for ill patients, usually in the household or hospital. Although smallpox is much less transmissible than measles, primary varicella, or influenza, secondary attack rates among unvaccinated contacts range from 37% to 88%. In certain cases, patients who are coughing can transmit large quantities of virus by aerosol. In Meschede, Germany, 17 persons on 3 floors of a hospital contracted smallpox from a patient admitted for a febrile illness presumed initially to be typhoid fever; this outbreak was ascribed to the patient's cough and the low relative humidity and air currents in the hospital.

At room temperature and relatively low humidity the virus survives in crusts from infected patients for as long as 16 weeks. Thus both fomite transmission from such items as bedsheets and blankets has been documented. A number of laundry workers who handled linens and blankets used by patients have developed disease. Disinfectants that are used for standard hospital infection control, such as hypochlorite and quaternary ammonium compounds, are effective for cleaning surfaces possibly contaminated with the virus.

Ideally only vaccinated persons should care for the patient. If there is an inadequate number of vaccinated individuals, vaccination of additional personnel should be done, immediately after which they are able to care for the patient. The long incubation period of variola infection allows the vaccine to modify the course of illness after exposure.

QUARANTINE

Smallpox was one of the standard internationally quarantinable diseases until its elimination, and it specifically remains on the US list of federally quarantinable diseases. Therefore, patients with suspected contact with smallpox patients could be detained by health authorities for monitoring. With options for vaccination postexposure, it is reasonable that any quarantine period might be limited on vaccination with appropriate postvaccination follow-up to ensure successful vaccination and interruption of disease transmission. Additionally, options such as home quarantine would be reasonable to consider, with additional vaccination of household members.

Monkeypox

HISTORY

The term "monkeypox" is a misnomer, based on the original isolation of the virus in 1958 from a colony of ill monkeys kept for research. While it has only been isolated once from a wild animal (a squirrel in the Democratic Republic of the Congo [DRC]), one or more species of rodents that inhabit the secondary forests of Central Africa are presumed to serve as the natural reservoirs. Monkeypox differs from variola in its ability to infect and cause illness outside of its reservoir species, and both non-human primates and humans develop clinical illness, which may prove fatal. Human monkeypox was not recognized as a distinct infection in humans until 1970 during efforts to eradicate smallpox, when the virus was isolated from a patient with suspected smallpox infection.

MICROBIOLOGY

Monkeypox virus is an orthopoxvirus in the same genus as variola and vaccinia. As with other orthopoxviruses, there appears to be significant cross-protection with vaccinia and variola infection. Two distinct geographic strains of the monkeypox virus exist. The Central African strain is more virulent, with mortality rates as high as 10%. The Western African strain lacks several genes compared to the Central African strain and causes less severe disease.

EPIDEMIOLOGY

Monkeypox has probably affected humans in endemic areas for millennia. Transmission from rodents to humans occurs from the handling of rodents used for bushmeat, as well as bites, scratches, and exposure to infected body fluids. Human-to-human transmission appears to be less efficient than for smallpox; however, it was seen to occur in up to 11.7% of household contacts of patients who had not received the smallpox vaccination. Household contacts and those caring for a monkeypox patient are at increased risk for acquiring infection.

Recently there have been outbreaks reported in several Central African countries. Waning immunity as well as increased dependence on hunting for food in areas devastated by civil war have been considered the most likely explanations for this increase. In 2003 an outbreak of human monkeypox (West African strain) occurred in the United States as the result of exposure to infected prairie dogs that had been housed close to rodents imported from Africa. There were 71 identified cases and no fatalities.

PATHOGENESIS

Disease pathogenesis is similar to that described for variola (above). After exposure by one of the routes noted above, the incubation period ranges from 9 to 13 days, shorter with either a larger inoculum or with percutaneous, as opposed to mucous membrane, exposure and accompanied by more severe disease manifestations.

CLINICAL MANIFESTATIONS

Based largely on sero-epidemiological studies in Africa, the majority of monkeypox infections are associated with mild nonspecific illness or are asymptomatic. Many of the clinical characteristics of human monkeypox infection mirror those of smallpox. Rash is preceded by a few days by fever, headache, myalgias, and lymphadenopathy affecting submental (causing jaw pain), cervical, and inguinal nodes. Enlarged lymph nodes are firm, tender, and sometimes painful. Rash often first appears on the face and quickly develops in a centrifugal distribution. Lesions can also involve mucous membranes, and oral lesions can cause difficulty with eating and drinking. The rash usually begins as macules and papules, which progress over approximately 2 weeks to vesicles and pustules. Similar to smallpox, all lesions evolve in the same stage of development, a critical differentiation from varicella (chicken pox). Pustules crust over after 1 to 2 weeks and then desquamate. The duration of illness is approximately 4–5 weeks from onset of the prodrome. Mortality rates from the Central African strain may be as high as 10%.

DIAGNOSIS

The diagnostic algorithm mentioned above for smallpox is useful in evaluating a possible case of monkeypox. History and clinical features aid in establishing the diagnosis, but definitive confirmation is established by virus isolation, real-time PCR, or immunofluorescent assay, all of which are done in a reference laboratory. Recognition of characteristic brick-shaped virions on electron microscopy (EM) distinguishes monkeypox from varicella, but the appearance on EM is identical to variola.

Varicella is the major disease in the differential, and distinguishing characteristics of monkeypox include lymphadenopathy and cutaneous lesions being in similar stages of development/healing. Additional vesiculopustular rash illnesses included in the differential are other herpetic infections, drug rash, syphilis, yaws, and scabies. Tanapox is another African poxvirus that causes a viral prodrome and skin lesions. Orf and bovine stomatitis can produce localized skin lesions but have a different appearance under EM.

TREATMENT

Tecovirimat, a recently licensed drug for treatment of smallpox, has activity against monkeypox. It has been shown to protect nonhuman primates from a lethal monkeypox challenge. See above discussion of use for smallpox. Brincidofovir also has the potential for activity against human monkeypox.

VACCINATION ISSUES

Vaccination against smallpox provides protection against other orthopoxvirus infections, including monkeypox. Whereas the degree of protection is less than complete, disease severity is significantly less in vaccinated individuals. In the US outbreak, 6 of 29 evaluated cases of symptomatic disease (24%) had received prior childhood smallpox vaccination. There was a trend toward milder disease in these individuals. Studies conducted in the DRC from 1981 to 1986 in the days following smallpox eradication showed that the attack rate of household members was significantly lower among those who had prior smallpox vaccination than among those without vaccination. Prior vaccination conferred 85% protection against monkeypox.

ISOLATION

Transmission of monkeypox is likely a rare event in the health care setting. The use of contact and airborne isolation precautions are recommended for any generalized vesicular rash of unknown etiology in which monkeypox and smallpox are in the differential diagnosis. Similar to variola, the virus is likely to survive for longer periods in low-humidity environments. Routine hospital cleaning agents are sufficient to kill monkeypox virus.

QUARANTINE

Monkeypox is not on the list of federally quarantinable diseases nor in the international health regulations. However, given its similarity to smallpox in clinical presentation, for individuals who have been exposed to someone with a smallpox-like illness, active monitoring or some restriction of movement might be considered until the symptomatic case is determined to be monkeypox rather than smallpox. Vaccination may be considered a potential option for exposed individuals, depending on the extent of presumed exposure.

CHAPTER 13

Henipaviruses and Other Miscellaneous Pathogens

SUSAN L. F. MCLELLAN

Introduction

The henipaviruses are a recently described genus of zoonotic viruses, two of which have been recognized to cause outbreaks in humans as well as animals. Although relatively rare, Nipah virus (NiV) and Hendra virus (HeV) both have the potential for significant economic impact due to epidemics in animal populations, as well as human disease with potential for person-to-person, including nosocomial, transmission. In humans, both diseases are highly lethal, and medical countermeasures are in very early stages of development. Outbreaks due to these viruses have been identified only in Australia and southern and southeast Asia; however, the animal reservoir, bats of the *Pteropodidae* family, have a wide distribution that includes Africa, and evidence for henipaviruses in bats has been documented as far as West Africa. A wide range of mammalian species can be infected experimentally with the henipaviruses and multiple animal models exist for research, but no wild reservoirs other than bats have been identified. Both Hendra and Nipah viruses are considered biosafety level 4 pathogens.

Nipah virus (NiV)

Nipah virus was first recognized as a cause of human disease after an outbreak in Malaysia in 1998–99. The outbreak of encephalitis was originally thought to be due to Japanese encephalitis, but in March 1999 a novel paramyxovirus was identified from the cerebrospinal fluid of an individual from Sungai Nipah village. This outbreak was associated with pigs and pig farming, and was transported to Singapore via infected carcasses. It is proposed that pigs raised in large-scale pig farms became infected by ingestion of fruit contaminated with bat saliva, as the reservoir fruit bats are found in proximity to the farms and frequently drop partially consumed fruit. There was very little evidence of person-to-person spread in the Malaysia/Singapore outbreak. The vast majority of cases were associated with direct contact with the pigs. Later outbreaks in Bangladesh and India, in contrast, have been associated primarily with consumption of date palm sap contaminated with bat excreta, and human-to-human transmission, including in health care facilities, has been a prominent concern. Other animals have also been found to be infected, including cows, goats, cats, and dogs. A significant outbreak in the Philippines occurred in 2014 in horses. Some transmission may have been associated with these domestic animals, including by ingestion of infected horsemeat. The virus is highly contagious among pigs, which produce copious secretions, with high morbidity rates but relatively low mortality.

Humans develop disease ranging from asymptomatic infection to severe encephalitis and death, although asymptomatic disease appears to be rare. A respiratory component is common, affecting approximately half of patients with severe neurologic signs, and exposure to respiratory secretions is the most likely means of person-to-person transmission. There may be some strain differences; for example, in the Malaysia outbreak, severe respiratory symptoms were much less common than in the subsequent Bangladesh and India outbreaks. The incubation period is described as 4–14 days, with initial fever, headache, vomiting, and sore throat, with or without respiratory symptoms such as cough or respiratory distress. In Bangladesh, significant frothing at the nose and mouth was described in late stages. In severe cases there is eventual development of lethargy and confusion with potentially rapid development of seizures and coma. If fatal, death occurs most commonly within 1–2 weeks. Case fatality rates have ranged from 40% to 75%. Higher rates were frequently found in settings where intensive care was not available or accessed. Among survivors of encephalitis, approximately 20% to 30% will suffer some neurologic sequelae. Additionally, there have been reports of relapse or late-onset encephalitis.

The diagnosis of NiV infection is made by immunohistochemistry, RT-PCR or conventional PCR of respiratory secretions, tissues, or cerebrospinal fluid, or serology by ELISA.

There are no approved vaccines or therapeutics for either of the henipaviruses. Vaccine trials in both livestock and humans are under way, as are trials of antivirals and antibody-based therapies.

Transmission, Infectivity, and Contagion. Most cases of Nipah virus disease in humans have been due to transmission from zoonotic hosts, either by contact with respiratory secretions (such as those from pigs) or other bodily fluids, or through ingestion of excreta (of bats in palm sap) or tissues of infected animals (pigs, horses). Infection of humans may also occur by ingestion of fruit contaminated by bats, but that association has not been demonstrated clearly.

Person-to-person transmission is clearly associated with close contact. Highest risk is associated with contact with persons who died (presumably with higher viral loads) and via contact with respiratory secretions and saliva. Handwashing and avoidance of the ill person have been associated with protection. The virus has also been isolated from urine, and has been recovered from sheets and towels. Epidemiologic investigation suggests that close exposure to saliva and respiratory secretions of an ill person presents a very high risk, and towels used by caregivers for more than one patient may act as fomites. During the Malaysia/Singapore outbreak, person-to-person spread was rare. This may have been due to both a lower rate of respiratory symptoms in patients and to relatively stronger infection control practices in homes and care facilities. Health care workers who reported blood and body fluid exposures to skin and mucous membranes, and even needlesticks, did not become infected. In Bangladesh, transmission to household care providers and nosocomial transmission to informal care providers and other patients was common, but transmission to health care workers was not. Epidemiologic and anthropologic studies suggest that within health care facilities most nursing care was given by friends and family rather than formal health care providers. Such care in homes and facilities provided multiple opportunities for exposure to respiratory secretions including cleaning; kissing, whispering to, and spoon-feeding the patient; and finishing food partially consumed by the ill patient, particularly at the end of life. Health care workers in Bangladesh who reported exposures did not have evidence of seroconversion. However, in some outbreaks in India, where more intensive care was provided (including nasogastric tubes and intubation) but infection control practices were poor, the risk to health care workers in facilities was higher. In at least one case, transmission was linked to the performance of funeral rites, which included cleaning of the orifices of the corpse, including the mouth and nasal cavities, without personal protective equipment (PPE). It is reasonable to assume that such activity would confer risk, but a pattern of funeral-related outbreaks has not been clearly observed. However, individuals involved in funeral rites are often the same persons who have been caregivers, so separating those risk factors is difficult.

It has also been recognized that some individuals appear to be "super-spreaders" and are responsible for a high proportion of secondary cases. Characteristics that define a super-spreader appear to be more related to host factors than to viral traits and may include viral load, underlying immune status, ability to produce secretions, and social status (high social status results in more contacts).

Need for Quarantine of Exposed Persons. Thus far, no serosurveys of persons without disease but with a history of exposure to known cases, have indicated a significant risk of asymptomatic infection. In addition, the risk of transmission is highest from patients who died, suggesting that severity of disease correlates with contagiousness. Respiratory secretions of patients with pulmonary symptoms appear to be the most common means of transmission. Hence, quarantine of asymptomatic exposed persons seems unlikely to provide benefit. Close surveillance of caregivers and close household contacts for the development of symptoms is reasonable, however, and has been implemented in previous outbreaks.

Isolation of Symptomatic Persons. Although the data is incomplete, available information suggests that direct contact with respiratory secretions and droplets from symptomatic patients are the major risk for person-to-person and nosocomial transmission. Significant nosocomial spread to persons with near, but not direct, contact in enclosed hospital settings, including to other patients and their caregivers, has been documented, although this typically occurs in the setting of recognized pulmonary symptoms and coughing without the use of personal protective measures. The epidemiology does not suggest airborne spread in general, but other paramyxoviruses such as measles can be transmitted in that manner, so that possibility exists, especially in the setting of aerosol-generating procedures.

Current recommendations from the World Health Organization (WHO) and Centers for Disease Control and Prevention (CDC) emphasize contact and droplet precautions. Most nosocomial transmission has occurred in settings with poor infection control practices, so determination of whether more aggressive measures are warranted is difficult.

WHO-supported Bangladeshi guidelines recommend isolation in a separate ward and barrier precautions including mask, gown, gloves, and shoe covers, with enforced hand hygiene. An N-95 mask is recommended for procedures with an aerosol risk such as intubation and suction. Eye protection is not mentioned. It should be noted that these guidelines are recommended in the setting of very minimal baseline infection control practices in many facilities of the country and would be difficult to achieve in some settings. In a more resourced setting, it would be reasonable to recommend eye protection be added for the care of a patient with any pulmonary symptoms.

Need for High-Level Isolation. Consideration of whether a patient should be treated in a specialized isolation unit is based on a combination of factors, including the infectivity of the pathogen (including infectious dose), case fatality rate, modes of transmission, availability of resources, and availability of medical countermeasures. Historical epidemiologic information can inform risk assessment but may not be applicable to highly resourced settings. In the case of Nipah virus, most nosocomial transmission has occurred in settings where even basic standard precautions were not available, and initiation of contact and droplet precautions would be expected to reduce transmission. However, options for medical countermeasures are limited, and this fact, combined with the high case fatality of NiV infection, might prompt the consideration of more stringent isolation conditions in highly resourced settings. Furthermore, in more highly resourced settings the likelihood of interventions that might aerosolize respiratory secretions is higher. The European Network of Infectious Diseases recommended airborne precautions at a minimum for "Hendra-like" viruses with the optimal situation involving high-level containment. An informal survey of clinicians working in high-level containment care (HLCC) units indicated that 44% would treat "Hendra-like" viruses in an HLCC unit; the balance favored either standard hospital setting or a case-by-case decision. Factors that would favor treatment in an HLCC unit would include copious respiratory secretions and potentially gastrointestinal secretions; there is little data to support shedding of virus in stool in humans, but it has been isolated from human urine and gastrointestinal fluids from bats. The need for invasive procedures such as intubation would also factor in the decision, as would severity of illness.

Termination of Isolation Precautions. There is very little data to guide the discontinuation of isolation precautions. However, data from one study suggests that viral shedding declines with the development of immunoglobulin M (IgM) antibodies, so it is probably reasonable to discontinue isolation as clinical condition improves and respiratory symptoms resolve.

Hendra virus (HeV)

Hendra virus (HeV), originally known as equine morbillivirus, was first identified in an outbreak in horses in 1994 in Queensland, Australia. Since then several other outbreaks have occurred in Australia, affecting more than 70 horses as of 2016. Only 7 cases in humans have been reported, 4 of which were fatal. All were in persons who had very close contact with sick horses, such as performing autopsies without appropriate PPE or very heavy exposure to secretions. There have been no human-to-human transmissions, and multiple other persons who had contact with ill horses did not develop disease. Illness in both humans and horses can include a severe respiratory syndrome that can progress to encephalitis. As with Nipah virus, fatal recrudescent neurologic disease has occurred.

Also, as with Nipah virus, diagnosis is typically made by RT-PCR, serology, viral isolation, or immunohistochemistry of tissues. No specific vaccine for humans exists; antiviral and antibody-based therapies are in early trials.

Considerations for Quarantine, Isolation, and Infection Control. Quarantine is not recommended for contacts of human or animal cases, and Australian infection control policy does not recommend restriction of movement for asymptomatic contacts. Given the lack of evidence for human-to-human transmission, and epidemiologic evidence suggesting that a heavy exposure is needed to result in human infection, there are few guidelines suggesting the need for high-level isolation. South Australian health guidelines recommend that persons infected with Hendra virus be restricted from work, childcare, day care, and school until well. Australian infection control guidelines recommend standard, contact, and droplet precautions for most care, with airborne precautions if aerosol-generating procedures are likely. Considerations for high-level isolation would be similar to those for NiV, with the caveat that human-to-human transmission appears to be less common than with NiV, and also acknowledging the limited number of human data from which to make recommendations.

Severe Fever with Thrombocytopenia Syndrome

Severe fever with thrombocytopenia syndrome virus (SFTSV) is a recently described Phlebovirus belonging to the *Bunyaviridae* family. It is transmitted by ticks, primarily *Haemaphysalis longicornis* but also *Rhipicephalus microplus*. The former feeds on domestic animals, and serosurveys of these animals have revealed seroprevalence rates of up to 75% in chickens, goats, cattle, and sheep. Wild animals have lower rates of seroprevalence. These zoonotic hosts may have no or mild symptoms but may act as amplifying hosts. A specific primary zoonotic reservoir has not been identified.

Disease in humans was first identified in China in 2007, and several outbreaks have occurred there as well as South Korea and Japan. Case fatality rates have been as high as 30%. Most cases occur in adult farmers, but human-to-human transmission has occurred, including in nosocomial settings. The incubation period, at least from person-to-person cases, has been described as 8–13 days. Clinical presentation of disease begins with fever, followed by development of leukopenia and thrombocytopenia and biochemical evidence of organ dysfunction. Diarrhea (including melena) and vomiting (including hematemesis) have been reported as significant; respiratory symptoms have been less prominent, although respiratory failure can occur as a component of multi-organ system failure.

Reviews of risk factors for human-to-human transmission suggest that direct exposure to blood or respiratory secretions is the most common route. Whether respiratory secretions uncontaminated by blood are infectious is unclear as most of the source patients had bloody secretions or coincident hematemesis. Contacts of patients who did not participate in close care of the ill person or in funeral preparations were less likely to develop disease. Investigation of one cluster suggested that contact with nonbloody secretions resulted in asymptomatic infection, whereas contact with bloody secretions was associated with symptomatic disease. In general, infected health care providers were not using full barrier precautions.

Considerations for Quarantine, Isolation, and Infection Control. At the current time there is no evidence for transmission from asymptomatic persons, whether with incubating disease or with asymptomatic infection. Quarantine measures have not been recommended for exposed persons. Isolation for persons with clinical disease should clearly include contact precautions, and droplet precautions including eye protection would be recommended for many ill patients, especially if producing copious bodily secretions. Airborne precautions would be appropriate for procedures expected to generate aerosols. Considerations for care in high-level containment would be similar to those for other hemorrhagic fevers, although the data so far suggest that transmission does not occur as easily as with the filoviruses. Factors in favor of a higher isolation level would include hemorrhagic manifestations, especially complicating gastrointestinal losses, and the need for high-intensity interventions.

Plague

Plague, caused by the bacterium *Yersinia pestis,* is not a new disease, and in the most common form (bubonic) is not considered a significant risk for nosocomial spread. However, nosocomial transmission has occurred with the pneumonic form. The last such reported case in the United States was in the early 20th century, but more recent episodes have been documented in less resourced areas.

Infection with *Y. pestis* most commonly occurs from the bite of an infected flea, but the blood and tissues of a patient can be infectious. Transmission from an individual with pneumonic plague typically follows a droplet pattern, although as with other pathogens, certain procedures may carry a risk of aerosolization, including manipulation of the respiratory tract and some autopsy procedures.

Existing guidelines for the management of plague recommend contact precautions, and droplet precautions until either the pneumonic form has been excluded or treatment has been ongoing for 72 hours. Airborne precautions are warranted for certain procedures. High-level isolation has not been employed typically for the care of patients with plague. Most nosocomial transmission has occurred before the diagnosis was determined and in the absence of personal protective measures. Options for therapy and postexposure prophylaxis exist (antibiotics), and vaccines are available, although not currently produced in the United States.

Extensively Drug-Resistant Tuberculosis

Infection with tuberculosis (TB) is well known to be a risk for health care workers and other individuals in health care facilities, especially in environments where rigid infection control measures are not in place. Presumably the risk is similar for extensively drug-resistant TB (XDR-TB), and increased incidence of multidrug-resistant TB (MDR-TB) and XDR-TB has been documented in health care workers in areas with a high prevalence. However, transmission of TB, including XDR-TB, is almost universally via the airborne route, with small suspended airborne particles inhaled into alveoli; droplet and direct contact, including to mucous membranes, are negligible risks. There is no evidence of failure of appropriate airborne precautions to prevent transmission of XDR-TB to health care workers once a case is diagnosed. In addition, medical countermeasures (antituberculous antimicrobials) do exist for treatment and postexposure prophylaxis, although the regimens are relatively complicated and of long duration. High-level isolation precautions have not typically been recommended. However, increased environmental controls such as appropriate ventilation, negative pressure, and use of germicidal ultraviolet light; availability of respirators; and rapid diagnosis and initiation of therapy are important to reduce nosocomial transmission to health care workers and other patients. Forcible quarantine has been utilized in public health practice in situations where individuals fail to adhere to their antituberculous regimens and therefore pose a public health risk to others. Decisions on how and when to do this generally occur at the local level, although there is now a federal quarantine center at the University of Nebraska Medical Center. How that might be used related to cases of tuberculosis remains to be determined.

Rabies

Rabies, caused by the rabies virus, is a disease resulting almost uniformly in death and with few reliable medical countermeasures available once symptoms have developed. However, rabies has not been documented to have been transmitted nosocomially, and, outside of organ transplantation, there is only one anecdotal report of possible human-to-human transmission in the literature. Transmission typically occurs via transdermal or mucous membrane exposure to saliva of infected animals. Similar exposure to neurologic tissue can theoretically result in infection as well. Acquisition by inhalation of aerosols of bat excreta has been proposed but never confirmed. There are effective pre- and postexposure vaccination strategies for health care workers who come in contact with potentially infectious material (primarily saliva); postexposure prophylaxis is not recommended for casual contact, including that involving blood, urine, or feces of an infected person or animal. Current experience does not support the need for care in an HLCC unit.

CHAPTER 14

Diseases Warranting Airborne Precautions

JONATHAN GREIN

There are only a few infections that warrant airborne isolation precautions in the conventional hospital setting: tuberculosis, measles, and varicella. While most patients with these diseases may not require hospitalization, airborne transmission of these pathogens has been described in hospital settings. Airborne isolation strategies (including well-ventilated rooms, negative room air pressure relative to the corridor, and use of respirators by health care workers) have been successful in mitigating transmission risk.

Tuberculosis

Tuberculosis (TB) is a chronic bacterial infection most commonly caused by *Mycobacterium tuberculosis*. TB infects a third of the world's population and is the single leading cause of death by an infectious agent. Humans are the only reservoir, and a third of infected patients are undiagnosed. Prior infection does not confer immunity. The highest TB incidence is in sub-Saharan Africa and Asia.

Infection of the lung or airway (e.g., larynx) allows aerosolization of bacilli with coughing or speaking. Inhalation of small infectious droplets (<5 microns) into alveoli leads to uptake by macrophages, which migrate outside the lung. A cell-mediated immune response takes 2–10 weeks and is usually effective in containing primary infection within granulomas.

Latent (asymptomatic) TB represents 90% of infections and reflects a small burden of bacilli contained within granulomas. Active disease develops in 10%, but more frequently in those with HIV or on TNF-alpha inhibitor therapy, and usually represents reactivation from prior infection. Typical pulmonary TB involves upper lobe cavitation associated with chronic cough, hemoptysis, fevers, unintentional weight loss, and/or night sweats. Atypical pulmonary involvement presents with lower lobe infiltrates (with or without cavitation), pleural effusions, and hilar lymphadenopathy and is more frequent in the immunosuppressed. Patients with extrapulmonary TB (e.g., vertebral involvement) should always be evaluated for pulmonary disease.

Diagnosis of TB remains a significant challenge. Both PPD skin testing and interferon-gamma release assays (IGRA) assess cell-mediated response to TB antigens and are used to diagnose latent TB with similar sensitivity, but false negative results occur in 20%.

Culture is the diagnostic gold standard but takes 3–8 weeks. Nucleic acid amplification tests (NAATs) can allow for rapid identification (i.e., hours) of TB and resistance mutations that predict multidrug-resistant (MDR) TB with sensitivity and specificity similar to culture.

Sputum smears allow rapid quantification of bacilli, the burden of which correlates with contagiousness. Approximately 10,000 bacilli/mL are required for smear positivity. A single sputum AFB smear is approximately 60% sensitive compared to culture; two additional smears increase sensitivity an additional 12%. Smear-negative, culture-positive patients represent 30–60% of pulmonary TB cases and are less infectious but still responsible for 10–20% of transmission events.

Standard treatment requires multidrug therapy for at least 6 months. MDR TB is defined as resistance to isoniazid and rifampin and is responsible for >450,000 infections/year; treatment relies on second-line agents that may be less reliable. Extensively drug-resistant (XDR) TB is additionally resistant to a fluoroquinolone and a second-line injectable drug and carries high mortality. Given the limited treatment options, high mortality rate, and public health implications, some experts advocate that patients hospitalized with XDR-TB be managed in a biocontainment unit (see chapter 13). Bacille Calmette-Guerin vaccine (BCG) is a live attenuated vaccine for tuberculosis that can reduce the severity of childhood TB infections, but it does not protect against primary infection or reactivation, making it marginally useful in limiting transmission.

KEY INFECTION PREVENTION CONCEPTS

TB is exhaled in small aerosol droplets from patients with symptomatic disease affecting the lungs or respiratory tract, particularly through coughing, sneezing, or talking. TB is not transmitted by large respiratory droplets or direct contact. Patients with latent TB or exclusive extrapulmonary involvement are not considered infectious with rare exception (such as aerosolization from a cutaneous TB infection). Ultraviolet light readily inactivates TB bacilli, making transmission in outdoor settings very inefficient.

Prolonged exposure to shared airspace is typically required for transmission. Transmission risk varies by case and depends on: (1) contagiousness of the patient; (2) burden of exposure; (3) host susceptibility; and (4) strain type. Patients are considered more contagious if they are sputum smear-positive, have an active cough, have cavitary lung disease on chest X-ray or involvement of the larynx, or are not on effective treatment. Factors affecting the burden of exposure include exposure duration, room size and ventilation, and cough-inducing procedures (such as bronchoscopy or intubation). Children, the immunocompromised, or those with a high exposure burden are more likely to develop active disease.

Health care workers (HCWs) are at higher risk of contracting TB than the general population, and unrecognized TB patients pose the highest risk to these workers. The annual HCW TB acquisition incidence varies from ~5% in low-income countries to 1% or less in high-income countries. A three-tiered approach significantly reduces HCW TB infection rates. Administrative controls aim to reduce the number of TB exposures and include a TB program that facilitates the prompt recognition and isolation of suspect TB patients. Engineering controls reduce the concentration of airborne TB and involve well-ventilated rooms for TB suspects (minimum 12 air exchanges/hour) with negative air pressure relative to the corridor. Finally, personal protective equipment (PPE) includes use of a respirator (such as a fit-tested N95 mask) to minimize TB inhalation.

Airborne isolation precautions should be used for inpatients suspected of pulmonary TB, including use of a well-ventilated negative-pressure airborne infection isolation room (AIIR) and respirator use. Outside the room, patients should wear a surgical mask to minimize spread of respiratory droplets. In patients determined unlikely to have TB, airborne isolation may be discontinued when three sputum samples, collected at least 8 hours apart with one early morning sample, are negative. NAAT performed on at least one sputum sample may reduce time to diagnosis.

For patients with confirmed TB, airborne isolation should be continued until three consecutive sputum smears are negative. Treatment of drug-susceptible TB rapidly reduces transmissibility over several days. However, since results of susceptibility testing take weeks, isolation should be continued until the patient has completed 2 weeks of treatment with signs of clinical improvement. Discharge home requires coordination with the local health department to ensure that treatment is continued and to evaluate household contacts.

Patients with suspected or proven MDR TB are managed more conservatively given the significant consequences of transmission. While inpatient, airborne isolation may be continued either for the entire treatment duration or until sputum cultures finalize as negative.

Exposure investigations emphasize identifying those with the highest exposure burden (e.g., household contacts or HCWs performing an aerosol-generating procedure) and at highest risk of developing active infection (e.g., children or the immunocompromised). Exposed contacts should have a baseline PPD or IGRA test and repeat testing 8 or more weeks after exposure. Treating those with conversions may reduce risk of active disease by 60%.

Measles

Measles virus (rubeola) is one of the most contagious human pathogens and was responsible for 2 million deaths annually prior to vaccine availability in 1963. Dramatic reductions in global measles incidence over the last several decades represent a tremendous public health achievement, though areas of endemic transmission remain, particularly in Africa and Asia.

Measles is caused by an enveloped RNA virus member of the *Paramyxoviridae* family. In endemic areas, 95% have been infected by age 15 years. Measles virus is transmitted through respiratory droplets and aerosols. Inhalation or direct inoculation of the upper respiratory tract with infectious virus leads to viral replication in respiratory epithelium, followed by spread to local lymphatic tissue, subsequent viremia, and involvement of a wide range of organs. A robust humoral and cellular immune response confers lifelong immunity.

KEY CLINICAL FEATURES

The incubation period is typically 10–14 days, though it may be longer in adults. Initial symptoms include a prodrome of fever, malaise, conjunctivitis, cough, and coryza. Koplik's spots (bluish or grey "grains of sand" on a red base frequently seen on the buccal mucosa) are pathognomonic and may develop prior to the rash. Low suspicion for measles and lack of clinician experience may contribute to misdiagnosis of measles as Kawasaki's disease, scarlet fever, infectious mononucleosis, parvovirus, or enterovirus.

The characteristic morbilliform (maculopapular) rash develops 2–4 days after initial prodrome symptoms and is usually present with fever. It begins at the hairline and spreads downward to the face, trunk, and then extremities, and may become confluent. The rash resolves in the same order it appeared and may desquamate. Transient leukopenia may occur. Most patients fully recover 7–10 days after symptom onset. Rash may be absent in immunocompromised patients. Treatment is supportive; vitamin A may reduce complications.

Complications occur in 30% of cases and are more common in the malnourished or immunosuppressed. These include pneumonia (primary or secondary bacterial infection) or sight-threatening ocular involvement. Additionally, neurologic complications include acute measles encephalitis (with or without a rash) or fatal subacute sclerosing panencephalitis that begins insidiously 7–10 years after infection. Functional immunosuppression may follow measles infection and increase risk for bacterial pneumonia or tuberculosis.

Diagnosis is often made clinically. Elevated IgM antibody titers are diagnostic of acute measles, though they may not be detectable until several days after rash onset. False negative and positive IgM results may occur. RT-PCR can detect measles directly from throat, nasopharyngeal, or urine samples within the first several days of rash onset.

KEY INFECTION PREVENTION CONCEPTS

Measles virus is highly transmissible through large respiratory droplets and smaller aerosols that may remain suspended in the air for up to 2 hours after the patient has left the area. Patients are considered infectious 4 days prior to the onset of rash, exacerbated by the cough of escalating prodromal symptoms. Rash onset heralds peak viral replication and the beginning of the adaptive immune response, though patients remain infectious for an additional 4 days.

Suspect measles patients should be masked and avoid waiting rooms; triage staff should be trained to promptly isolate suspect patients. Inpatients should be placed in negative-pressure isolation rooms; outpatients should be seen as the last case of the day and use alternative entrances. Health care providers caring for measles patients should have evidence of measles immunity, although respirators (i.e., N95 masks) are still recommended to prevent breakthrough infections.

All eligible HCWs should demonstrate evidence of measles immunity. Two doses of vaccine confer 99% protection. Breakthrough infections can occur but are less severe and are less infectious. Given its ease of transmissibility, a high level of population immunity is required to interrupt transmission.

Postexposure management consists of vaccination for those nonimmune. Given that measles is one of only a few infections that may be contagious prior to symptom onset, quarantine of exposed individuals can be considered for those who are nonimmune (such as those who decline or have contraindications to vaccination). The CDC defines evidence of immunity as written documentation of one or more measles vaccine after age 1 (two or more for high-risk individuals such as HCWs), lab evidence of immunity or prior measles infection, or born before 1957. Measles vaccination given within 72 hours of exposure may provide some protection. Immune globulin should be offered to patients at high risk of complications or with contraindication to vaccine (including pregnant women, infants <12 months, or immunocompromised patients). Nonimmune HCWs should not return to work through the duration of the incubation period, regardless of prophylaxis given.

Measles only infects humans, is vaccine preventable, is not transmitted by asymptomatic carriers, and confers lifelong immunity; these factors make it an attractive target for global eradication.

Varicella and Zoster

Varicella zoster virus (VZV) is an enveloped DNA virus and member of the *Herpesviridae* family that is ubiquitous and exclusive to humans. Primary varicella infection is characterized by a self-limited febrile rash syndrome (chicken pox), leading to viral latency and reactivation later in life as zoster (shingles). In temperate climates, primary infection is most common in children younger than 10 years.

Primary infection occurs when a susceptible individual inhales aerosolized virus, infecting respiratory mucosa. Viremia with infected T-lymphocytes may precede rash onset by up to 10 days and disseminates infection to the skin and other organs. Robust cell-mediated immunity develops, which can be lifelong, although mild breakthrough infections do occur.

KEY CLINICAL FEATURES

The symptoms of primary varicella begin 14–16 days (range 10–21) following exposure. A pruritic rash is often the first symptom in children, although a mild prodrome (low-grade fever, malaise, and headache) may precede rash onset by 1–2 days. The rash rapidly evolves from maculopapular to vesicular ("dewdrops on a rose petal"), then pustular before scabbing over. Multiple stages of evolution are present at any given time and may involve the entire body, including mucosal surfaces. Skin lesions will scab within 1 week, heralding the end of infectivity.

Complications of primary varicella infection are infrequent but are more likely to occur in the immunocompromised, neonates, or adults. These include secondary bacterial infection of the lung or skin (e.g., group A *Streptococcus*), severe varicella (prolonged viral replication), or encephalitis. Primary varicella during pregnancy is associated with potentially life-threatening varicella pneumonia, and if it develops during the first two trimesters of pregnancy can cause severe congenital defects. Neonatal varicella is associated with high mortality (30%).

Zoster incidence becomes more common after age 50 and reflects waning cell-mediated immunity. It typically presents as a unilateral painful vesicular rash along a single (or neighboring) neurologic dermatome(s). Disseminated zoster may occur in the immunosuppressed and involves noncontiguous dermatomes.

Diagnosis is often clinical. PCR of vesicular fluid is highly sensitive. Direct immunofluorescence performed on cells from an active (non-crusted) vesicle may provide a rapid diagnosis. Viral culture has lower yield than PCR. Serology can be used to screen for immunity but has limited utility in diagnosing active infection.

Treatment of primary varicella is primarily supportive. Concomitant aspirin use is associated with Reyes syndrome and should be avoided. Acyclovir (or its analogues) is recommended for patients with severe disease or at increased risk for complications. IV acyclovir is recommended for immunosuppressed patients or those with severe disease and is most beneficial when given within the first 24 hours after rash onset. Acyclovir is recommended to reduce severity and duration of zoster symptoms.

KEY INFECTION PREVENTION CONCEPTS

Transmission of VZV within health care settings is well recognized. Although all forms of VZV are potentially infectious, primary varicella is considered the most infectious with a 90% attack rates for susceptible household contacts.

Patients with primary varicella are considered infectious 1–2 days prior to rash onset until all lesions are crusted, and the degree of infectivity correlates with the severity of skin involvement. Virus is aerosolized from vesicular fluid in skin lesions and possibly from the respiratory tract and may spread through either the airborne route or through direct contact. Both airborne and contact precautions are recommended until all lesions have crusted. All HCWs should demonstrate immunity (documentation of 2 doses of vaccine or confirmatory serology), and only those with confirmed immunity should care for patients with primary varicella.

Isolation precautions are still recommended for immune HCWs given the possibility of breakthrough infections.

Zoster is common in health care settings and is significantly less infectious than primary varicella. Transmission may occur from direct contact with active skin lesions and may cause primary varicella in susceptible persons. For otherwise immunocompetent patients with localized zoster, standard precautions should be used. Aerosolization and airborne transmission from localized zoster lesions has been reported (rarely) in health care settings, emphasizing the importance of covering active lesions. Patients with disseminated zoster should be managed like primary varicella. Immunosuppressed patients with localized zoster are at higher risk for disseminated infection and should also be managed like primary varicella until disseminated infection has been ruled out.

Managing exposures includes rapid assessment of immunity in exposed individuals and administration of vaccine or varicella-zoster immune globulin (VZIG) to those susceptible. As people may become infectious prior to symptom onset, quarantine of individuals who are exposed but nonimmune may be considered, particularly for people in contact with those at risk for VZV complications (such as health care workers). The definition of exposure in hospital settings includes face-to-face contact for at least 5 minutes or presence in the same room for at least 1 hour. Exposed but immune HCWs should undergo daily monitoring for symptoms between postexposure days 8–21 and immediately removed from patient care if symptoms develop. Nonimmune HCWs should be removed from patient care areas during postexposure days 8–21; vaccination within 5 days of exposure may reduce disease severity. Exposed nonimmune individuals at risk for severe disease who have contraindication to vaccination should receive VZIG as soon as possible, within 10 days of exposure.

Vaccination (live attenuated Oka strain) is safe and has reduced primary varicella incidence by 97% in the United States. Vaccination leads to subclinical infection and subsequent latency similar to wild type virus, but the Oka strain is very unlikely to cause rash or secondary transmission. Zoster vaccines (live virus and inactivated subunit) are now available.

CHAPTER 15

Miscellaneous Diseases Subject to Quarantine

THEODORE J. CIESLAK

US Presidential Executive Order 13295 designates eight infectious conditions as candidates for federally imposed quarantine. Five of these conditions are already covered in chapters 10–14 of this manual. Here we address the remaining diseases: cholera, diphtheria, and yellow fever.

Cholera

Cholera, caused by the gram-negative bacterium *Vibrio cholerae*, is characterized by profuse watery diarrhea. The volume of stool output among cholera victims can be so great that voluntary oral fluid intake is inadequate to keep up with losses. In the absence of ongoing fluid replacement with intravenous fluids or oral rehydration solutions, patients can succumb to dehydration and electrolyte imbalances. Although the average infectious dose of ~100 million organisms is high in comparison to many other infectious diseases described in this manual, one gram of stool from a person infected with cholera may contain trillions of organisms, thus enhancing the potential for disease spread. Cholera is typically acquired as a result of poor environmental hygiene and consumption of feces-contaminated water, rather than direct person-to-person transmission. The vast majority of cholera cases occur in resource-poor areas of sub-Saharan Africa and in the Ganges

River delta of Bangladesh and eastern India, where fecal matter often contaminates drinking water sources.

Isolation. Transmission in health care settings is rare and can be avoided by simple handwashing and meticulous attention to the proper handling of human waste and contaminated linens. For these reasons, cholera patients would not likely require high-level isolation in an inpatient setting.

Quarantine. The quarantine of asymptomatic individuals in order to stop a cholera outbreak would also be unnecessary in most instances. While experience in the 19th century, when ships were quarantined in New York's East River near Bellevue Hospital, attests to the effectiveness of such measures, the utility of simpler methods to reduce disease spread, such as those taken by John Snow (who legend has it halted a cholera outbreak in London by removing a water pump handle), argue against its necessity in most cases. Nonetheless, cholera remains subject to federal quarantine in the United States and had long been one of the World Health Organization's (WHO) few quarantinable diseases. It is thus conceivable that quarantine might be employed as an adjunct to other hygiene-based control measures should a cholera outbreak occur. As humans are the only reservoir of cholera (although the causative organism survives *ex vivo* in salt water), the disease presents an eradication target. Future efforts aimed at mopping up remaining pockets of disease might include human quarantine. The short incubation period of cholera (2 hours to 5 days) means that such quarantine would likely be limited in duration but also challenging to implement effectively in a rapidly expanding outbreak.

Finally, vaccination might be offered to health care workers and close contacts of cholera victims as an adjunct to hygiene-based measures. Vaxchora®, licensed in the United States in 2016, offers short-term protection against *V. cholera* strain O1 (the historical cause of cholera in Africa and Asia) to a majority of recipients. It does not protect against other cholera strains, including *V. cholera* strain O139, found in the Americas.

Diphtheria

Diphtheria, caused by the gram-positive bacillus *Corynebacterium diphtheriae*, most often presents as a severe pharyngeal or laryngeal infection. Victims risk airway obstruction and hypoxia caused by edema and necrosed infected tissues in the posterior pharynx known as pseudomembranes. A potent toxin produced by the organism can also cause fatal myocarditis and other complications. Cutaneous infection can occasionally occur. Diphtheria is generally transmitted person to person through direct contact with nasopharyngeal secretions or droplets. The incubation period is 1–10 days. In colonial times, diphtheria was a major cause of childhood mortality. The appearance of diphtheria, which is extremely contagious via respiratory droplets, in a village could threaten its entire pediatric population. Extraordinarily effective vaccines against the toxin, available since 1921, as well as antibiotics, have nearly eliminated diphtheria from most developed nations. Its propensity for a rapid return, however, is illustrated by outbreaks that occurred in the 1990s in all 15 republics of the former Soviet Union following the dissolution of the latter and a consequent breakdown in public health infrastructure and immunization efforts.

Isolation. The institution of droplet precautions would constitute adequate isolation for a hospitalized patient with diphtheria.

Quarantine. While quarantine was a mainstay of diphtheria control in the pre-antibiotic era, it would not likely be necessary in most cases today, although short-term confinement of close contacts of diphtheria patients might be utilized to facilitate administration of prophylactic antitoxin. It is also conceivable that public health authorities might, in the face of a diphtheria outbreak, invoke quarantine in the management of unvaccinated individuals, vaccine refusers, other noncompliant persons, and potential super-spreaders. Like cholera, diphtheria has no animal reservoir and presents an eradication target. Limited quarantine might have a role in such efforts in the future.

Yellow Fever

Yellow fever is a disease of humans and other primates and is caused by a flavivirus transmitted by *Aedes* mosquitoes. In roughly 85% of patients, the illness is self-limited and presents, following a 3–6 day incubation period, with headache and high fever. While these symptoms typically resolve within a few days, a secondary phase occurs in a minority of patients. This phase involves gastrointestinal signs and symptoms (vomiting, epigastric pain, and jaundice) as well as a bleeding diathesis, manifest by hematemesis, melena, hematuria, ecchymoses, and other signs of clotting dysfunction and hemorrhage. The scleral icterus often seen at this point lends the disease its name, and renal insufficiency as well as cardiovascular instability are common in this later stage. Viremia is usually present only during the first three days of illness, and while the disease is not directly transmissible from person to person, viremic patients risk infecting local mosquitoes.

Isolation. Because the disease is not generally transmissible except via these arthropod vectors, standard precautions are adequate in managing hospitalized patients. A licensed vaccine, YF-Vax®, is offered to (and sometimes required of) persons in the United States traveling to endemic areas. Various other yellow fever vaccines are available in a number of foreign countries, although shortages of vaccine have hampered immunization efforts. Because of the lack of person-to-person transmission, vaccines would likely be of little benefit to health care workers in nonendemic areas.

Quarantine. *Aedes* mosquitoes are found throughout the tropics, the subtropics, and in many parts of the temperate world; therefore, concern for reintroducing yellow fever to geographic areas from which it had been eliminated might prompt quarantine of a patient.

Other Diseases

In the past, quarantine has been used for patients feared to be harboring polio, typhoid fever, typhus, anthrax, leprosy, and scarlet fever. None of these diseases remain on current lists of quarantinable conditions and all can be controlled by far less restrictive means. Typhus and anthrax are not transmitted from person-to-person, while polio and typhoid are contagious only via the fecal-oral route. Leprosy has nearly been eliminated from the developed world and is only minimally communicable. Scarlet fever has become a relatively trivial disease in the antibiotic era. Nonetheless, as humanity enters the final stages of polio eradication and leprosy elimination, it remains possible that quarantine could be ordered in isolated circumstances (to vaccine refusers, in the case of polio, for instance). Conversely, as old diseases are eradicated, new ones will continue to emerge. Consequently, the list of diseases subject to quarantine will likely evolve further over time.

CHAPTER 16

Special Populations

Pediatric and Obstetric Patients

THEODORE J. CIESLAK
JOHN P. HORTON
MARK G. KORTEPETER

Pediatrics

A well-known mantra of pediatric medicine reminds us that "children are not simply little adults." In fact, children differ from adults in myriad ways, many of which potentially impact their susceptibility and response to infectious diseases, as well as the ability to care for them once they become ill.

Anatomic and Physiologic Differences. Children have an increased surface-area-to-volume ratio as compared to adults. This results in the potential for greater transcutaneous heat and fluid loss and necessitates more meticulous attention to fluid and electrolyte balance among ill children. Similarly, it results in a greater susceptibility to percutaneous absorption of noxious substances (such as chemicals, toxins, and radiation). These effects are exacerbated further by children's thinner and less well keratinized epidermis, and less subcutaneous tissue and fat. Furthermore, a child's head contributes a greater proportion of his or her mass and surface area; a newborn infant's head is 50% of its ultimate adult mass, while its body is only 5% of its ultimate mass. This is problematic in that the head is quite vascular and even more susceptible to heat loss than the remainder of the body. In addition, the head often cannot be fully covered in order to mitigate against this heat loss.

Children have an increased organ-to-body-mass ratio, making them more susceptible to traumatic organ injury. They have an increased minute ventilation, further compounding the problem of fluid loss, as well as increasing their exposure to noxious airborne particles and infectious agents. They have an immature blood-brain barrier, facilitating the entry of substances (and potentially microbes) into the central nervous system. Finally, they have more rapidly dividing cells, rendering them more susceptible to the effects of radiation.

Developmental Considerations. Myriad developmental considerations affect a child's susceptibility to infection. Children have large and complex social networks, with high numbers of interpersonal contacts. Moreover, they are housed in schools and day care centers where they are more likely than adults to contract and spread infectious diseases. They also engage in high-energy activity and live "closer to the ground," making them particularly susceptible to contracting fomite-borne diseases; this susceptibility is further heightened by their tendency to place objects (fomites) in their mouths. While all of these factors would seem to increase a child's susceptibility, it should be noted that only 9–18% of victims of previous Ebola outbreaks were children, despite children making up roughly 50% of the people living in afflicted African nations. While it is possible that this reflects some inherent resistance to Ebola virus disease (EVD), it is more likely that children simply have less contact with infected persons (through caregiving roles and funereal preparations, for example). Notably, however, the most recent outbreak in North Kivu, Democratic Republic of the Congo, has been unusual in the higher percentage of infected children and mothers than in the past.

Similarly, developmental considerations affect a child's ability to accept care and to respond to caregivers. Young children are often unable to cooperate with care, to follow the instructions of caregivers and public safety personnel, to flee the scene of a disaster, and to distinguish fantasy from reality. As such, caregivers in personal protective equipment (PPE) may be especially frightening, and children may tug and pull at PPE, thus endangering those caregivers. They may also be more prone to the development of posttraumatic stress disorder (PTSD) than adults.

Pathologic Differences. Certain diseases produce different manifestations in children than they do in adults. Children with EVD are uniformly febrile, although only 16% exhibit hemorrhage. And, while respiratory and gastrointestinal symptoms are common among childhood EVD patients, central nervous system manifestations are rare. These factors combine to yield a clinical presentation in children that closely resembles influenza. Lassa fever has a mortality rate of 27% among symptomatic children, higher than that seen in adults. Moreover, congenital Lassa is nearly 100% fatal and presents a unique manifestation in infants, called "swollen baby syndrome," which has a mortality rate of approximately 75%.

Smallpox also poses unique challenges for children. While older adults may possess some residual immunity from decades-old vaccinations, today's children are uniformly unimmunized. Any attempt to ramp up an immunization campaign (in the face of a serious bioweapons threat, for example) would be hampered by an increased risk of vaccinial encephalitis among children compared with adults, as well as a risk of fatal fetal vaccinia among pregnant women. Pediatric plague victims may be more prone to digital necrosis (related to disseminated intravascular coagulation) than adults, owing to their smaller blood vessels, and to the development of plague meningitis. Finally, pediatric tuberculosis patients are more likely than their adult counterparts to develop life-threatening disease manifestations such as tuberculous meningitis and disseminated tuberculosis.

Therapy and Policy Considerations. Many therapeutic and political factors have the potential to affect the care of children with highly hazardous communicable diseases (HHCDs). Certain medications that might be used to treat adults are contraindicated in children, are unfamiliar to pediatric caregivers, or are unavailable in liquid preparations. Child-sized equipment is less widely available than is comparable adult equipment, and fewer personnel are trained in its use. Finally, pediatric-specific airborne infection isolation and high-level containment care (HLCC) beds are rare, pediatric-specific doctrine is sparse, and the conduct of research (and use of investigational drugs) is often more difficult in children.

During the 2014–16 West Africa outbreak, the HLCC units in the United States or Western Europe were not required to care for any pediatric patients with confirmed EVD; however, 18% of EVD patients in Guinea were children. Therefore, the care of pediatric patients in HLCC units should be a routine part of preparations. Several aspects need to be considered in such planning, including developing age-stratified stock lists for infants, toddlers, children, and adolescents; stockage of age- and size-appropriate pediatric equipment; pediatric-specific training and exercise scenarios for unit staff. A number of challenges must be considered to ensure the success of appropriate planning, as follows:

Parental Presence. Pediatric medicine embraces the concept of family-centered care, wherein parents are encouraged to participate actively in caring for their hospitalized child. In many instances (especially in the developing world), such participation is often expected, with parents or other family members providing many aspects of daily care, such as feeding, dressing, toileting, nursing, and comforting their child. However, appropriately addressing the possibility of parental presence at the bedside creates one of the most vexing problems encountered when caring for a child in an HLCC unit.

Therefore, it is imperative for facilities providing HLCC to children to have policies that address the presence of parents in a child's hospital room if they are infected with an HHCD, in addition to the other issues noted below. The policies should articulate which, if any, circumstances would allow parents to enter the HLCC unit and patient room, and should ideally be stratified by age, developmental status, medical condition, and pathogen. Such policies that limit parental presence, developed in advance of an admission, might prove especially beneficial in situations involving a highly contagious child, where parents feel familial or personal pressure to do so, but at the same time may be uncomfortable interacting with their child.

Currently, many HLCC experts advocate against allowing parents entry into an EVD-infected child's room. In addition to the potential risks of infection spread for those parents, the significant amount of training required in order for parents to don and doff PPE safely and properly would not be practical. Moreover, even a cooperative parent who has been well trained presents a potential risk to other personnel in the unit who are required to then monitor the parent to guard against inadvertent breaks in infection control while at the same time attending to the child. The confined space in most HLCC units makes such monitoring particularly difficult, especially when breaks in infection control technique and protocol violations might go undetected by nursing and other personnel in the unit who are focused on the well-being and care of a very ill child. Furthermore, in such a confined setting, additional nonessential personnel may increase the risk of falls, sharps injuries, PPE snags, and other inadvertent breaches.

There are numerous other considerations that argue for a cautious approach regarding parental presence. Once allowed entry to a child's room, parents might fail to recognize the gravity of potential symptoms or breaches in protocol, or may be reluctant to report them for fear of being excluded. Moreover, any parent who has a breach and must be placed under quarantine (or, worse, isolation if they become ill with the disease in question) loses the flexibility to care for other family members, thus increasing stress and adversely impacting the family's general well-being. Finally, nursing personnel typically wear PPE for 2–4 hour shifts, whereas parents may wear such garb for extended periods of time, increasing the burden on them and the staff who must monitor them. More time in PPE increases the risk of fatigue-induced mistakes.

Although many experts believe the risks of parental presence in the room of a child infected with EVD (or other viral hemorrhagic fever) outweigh its benefits, the possibility of allowing such presence under certain conditions has been raised, depending on the causative agent, a child's clinical status (i.e., whether "wet," with significant vomiting, diarrhea, or hemorrhage, or "dry"), the child's age and developmental status, and other aspects.

Whether limitations on parental presence should be applied to highly hazardous diseases that spread primarily by the airborne route, such as severe acute respiratory syndrome (SARS), Middle East respiratory syndrome (MERS), and novel influenza, is somewhat more controversial. The PPE ensembles needed to limit airborne transmission of such diseases are typically less burdensome than those required for managing EVD cases, and Centers for Disease Control and Prevention (CDC) guidelines already allow for family members and visitors to utilize N-95 respirators.

Use of video monitors to allow teleparenting as well as other technology solutions can help bridge the gap left by parental exclusion, although they are an admittedly inferior substitute for direct parental interaction. We recommend that parents be allowed to locate near the HLCC unit in a private, dedicated room, which allows ready access to telemonitoring equipment, therefore providing them nearly uninterrupted access to their child.

Cohorting. One of the primary concerns behind barring a parent from an infected child's room is the concern that the parent will contract the disease from their child. If the parent is already infected, such concerns no longer apply. In fact, EVD (and many other highly hazardous pathogens) typically spread to susceptible children from an adult household member. Therefore, the possibility exists that an infected child might reasonably be cohorted and cared for in the same room as their adult relative (or infected sibling). Resource constraints may require such a strategy in developing nations; however, we recommend against it in most cases. Both the child and parent may experience varying severity of disease or progress along differing disease time courses, making clinical management and psychological well-being of patients problematic in a cohort environment. For example, a parent who is improving clinically may witness the demise of his/her child (or vice versa), which could pose potential risks to themselves, as well as HLCC unit personnel. Temporary cohorting may be appropriate or unavoidable in the case of PUIs, if the family members have already been in close contact for extended periods, as long as we recognize the need to separate them if one individual rules in for disease while the others do not. Cohorting might also be appropriate when multiple family members are improving, but not yet ready for discharge. For any infant PUI born to an infected mother, the infant should be managed as if infected until infection can be ruled out definitively. Fathers and other uninfected potential caretakers should generally be excluded from contact with such a newborn, until the infant can be determined not to be infected.

Breastfeeding. Ebola virus is secreted in the breast milk of EVD-infected lactating mothers, and it remains present for some time after recovery. Consequently, and in line with CDC guidance, we recommend mothers with EVD should avoid breastfeeding. Although we do support breast pumping for relief of engorgement, expressed breast milk from EVD-infected mothers should be managed as a category A infectious substance. There may be other options that can be individualized with other pathogens, depending on their known potential to be secreted in breast milk. For example, with SARS, virus has not been isolated from breast milk, although antibodies to the virus can be found in recovering mothers. This raises the possibility that breastfeeding could actually be beneficial to the infant in the later stages of maternal disease.

Staffing. Having pediatric and neonatal nursing staff directly involved in caring for children with HHCDs is important; however, HLCC units employ multiple staffing models. Some favor using intensive care unit and emergency room nurses in a primary role, with support from pediatric and neonatal nurses, while others reverse those roles. In either case, the staffing ratios might need to exceed the 3:6 staff/patient model used by HLCC units in 2014 for adults, due to the need for the presence of a health care worker (HCW) in a child's room at all times and the extra staff potentially required to hold, comfort, or distract children undergoing procedures.

Staff Protection. Chapter 8 of this manual provides general advice on the use of PPE. However, when caring for young children, HLCC staff may choose to use supplements to their PPE, such as a cloth surgical gown, as an extra measure of protection against the possibility that an agitated, flailing toddler might rip or displace their underlying PPE. Any such modifications must weigh the potential benefits against the added heat stress associated with extra clothing and the impact this heat stress might have on further limiting HCW time spent on the unit in PPE. Despite its potential to interfere with play therapy and other therapeutic interactions between patients, their families, and caregivers, chemical sedation may be a necessary component of the management of a frightened, flailing toddler or child in certain situations and may be necessary to ensure both staff and patient safety. Similarly, physical restraint may occasionally be necessary in the HLCC setting, although we acknowledge that it is controversial. Its use should, consequently, be minimized, and it should be employed only in conjunction with other modalities such as chemical sedation, behavioral management, and parental assurance (via tele-technology).

Child Life. Therapeutic play is an important modality in the care of pediatric patients. Child life professionals and pediatric occupational therapists are invaluable in fostering the appropriate environment for such play to take place. Safety concerns will dictate whether such specialists should be kept from a child's room in most cases; however, exceptions might be made if such specialists are fully integrated into the HLCC unit care team, and if they participate in regular training alongside this team. In other situations, there are ways play therapy can be supported through using video teleconferencing or providing advice on play therapy to nurses and other members of the HLCC care team.

Toys play an obvious important role in a child's life, and they may help a child understand and cope with their time in the unique confines of an HLCC unit. For example, Texas Children's Hospital has designed a teddy bear garbed in PPE analogous to that worn by caregivers. Nonetheless, toys present an infection control risk in an HLCC unit, and any toys that enter the unit should, in most cases, be destroyed on the child's discharge. Theoretically, toys that can be autoclaved might be returned to a child; however, this might prove a logistical challenge, because it necessitates that a unit has an in-suite or on-campus autoclave and dedicated sterilization cycle. Having duplicate toys presents an alternative solution; for example, one teddy bear is destroyed while an identical duplicate is "discharged" home with the recovered child.

Reintegration. Children face numerous physical, emotional, and psychosocial stressors in the hospital environment, which are exacerbated when they are denied direct contact with parents and family. Not only do children suffer the direct effects of HHCDs, which often involve lengthy hospitalization, painful medical procedures, and prolonged recovery periods, but family members, friends, schoolmates, teachers, and others fearing contagion may treat survivors with suspicion. In addition to its negative effects on learning and psychosocial development, prolonged school absence may contribute to a sense of alienation from classmates. Flashbacks, which have been reported commonly among adult survivors of EVD, may amplify feelings of helplessness, hopelessness, and estrangement. Other aspects may exacerbate these problems, especially the death of parents or siblings, which commonly occurs among African children surviving with EVD.

For the reasons we have noted, it is paramount for facilities to have a coordinated approach to managing a child's treatment, recovery, and transition from the HLCC unit to a recuperative setting, and ultimately to complete family, school, and social reintegration. During a child's hospitalization, planning for such reintegration should begin as early as possible, and chances of success can be improved with assistance from child life providers, social workers, and child psychologists/psychiatrists.

Obstetrics

Every medical facility should include planning for the pregnant patient with an infectious disease. Preplanning for pregnancy contingencies includes responding to:

- Ectopic pregnancy
  - ◉ Bleeding with acute need to operate
  - ◉ Stable with potential options of medical therapy
- Miscarriage
  - ◉ Stable missed abortion
  - ◉ Incomplete abortion with bleeding
- Pregnancy without need to deliver
  - ◉ Previable
  - ◉ Viable
- Pregnancy with need to deliver fetus
  - ◉ Vaginal delivery
  - ◉ Cesarean delivery

Considering each of the above scenarios will generate significant dialogue about how to render care for a pregnant patient safely, or help determine what precautions are needed if delivery or surgery were to occur. Most important in the planning is the inclusion of all medical teams that might support a response, including obstetrics, maternal fetal medicine, neonatology, anesthesia, and nursing from all divisions with further consideration of the support staff such as respiratory therapy. Hospital ethics committees may be worth consulting as part of the planning process when considering the above scenarios to allow for expediting responses if and when a clinical case presents.

When considering pregnancy in the face of HHCDs, one must immediately bear in mind two things. First are the new potential sources of infectious pathogens including placental tissue, amniotic fluid and sac, and fetal sources. The second is to remember that any pregnant patient can transition from being dry to having copious liquid contamination from bodily fluids within moments as infection can increase the rate of miscarriage or preterm delivery. With rupture of amniotic membranes, amniotic fluid will continuously leak from the uterus until delivery of products of conception occurs. Large amounts of bleeding may occur with the delivery of products of conception with either a fetus of viable gestational age or miscarriage of an early gestational fetus. Infection may also increase the likelihood for uterine bleeding.

The response to postpartum hemorrhage or postmiscarriage bleeding should be practiced, and pharmacologic agents to aide in the treatment of bleeding need to be available on any unit considering care of the pregnant patient. These agents include but are not limited to carboprost, methylergonovine, misoprostol, and Pitocin. Each of them have optimal clinical use in the setting of postpartum hemorrhage, but some have side effects that should be considered. For example, carboprost can increase bowel motility resulting in diarrhea, potentially leading to a greater amount of infectious fluids.

Response to other common obstetric emergencies such as eclamptic seizure or fetal distress should be incorporated into response planning and practice to ensure expedited care when the need arises. It should be noted that fear of the pregnant patient should be directly addressed with all staff. The fear of harming the fetus or of the increased risk of infection has led to failure to act or a delay in care. Staff should be empowered and know that most protocols for the infected and contagious adult should carry on as planned even in the setting of pregnancy. Antibiotic choices may vary somewhat, and added precautions may be needed; however, pregnancy should not limit care. Most radiographic imaging techniques are reasonable to perform if the patient has emergent needs, with only a few techniques absolutely contraindicated, such as MRI with gadolinium contrast.

Reproductive goals should be discussed prior to discharge with all patients to provide appropriate counsel on potential future risks of transmission. The potential for sexual transmission and prevention measures should be communicated clearly to all patients of any gender, which should include discussion of contraception as a part of patient care plans, if desired, in the individual's reproductive goals.

CHAPTER 17

Laboratory Operations

PETER C. IWEN
VICKI L. HERRERA

Background

Laboratory safety represents one of the more difficult challenges associated with isolation and quarantine care. In these situations, laboratory managers and the isolation/quarantine team must balance the safety of laboratorians and health care workers with the ability to provide diagnostic and other clinical laboratory data that may be critical for clinical or public health decisions. With appropriate planning, both considerations can be adequately addressed.

An asymptomatic individual placed in quarantine following exposure to a high-risk pathogen may not require laboratory support during the infectious agent's incubation period. Exceptions might include serological testing to assess the individual's immune status, bloodwork to assess response to an experimental vaccine or other postexposure prophylactic, or baseline assessment of a number of parameters (blood counts, chemistries, liver functions, banked serology) for future comparison if illness were to occur. Additionally, an asymptomatic person in quarantine may need some laboratory support for an underlying condition that requires routine monitoring (i.e., the monitoring of glucose levels in a diabetic patient or the exclusion of other potential comorbid events). For most highly hazardous communicable diseases (HHCDs), specimens from exposed patients without symptoms can be handled in a standard bio-safety level 2 clinical laboratory using routine biosafety practices without enhanced precautions.

Once a person becomes symptomatic or is suspected of being capable of shedding infectious agent, the risk calculation changes and their disease becomes potentially communicable. They are then placed in isolation and reclassified as a person under investigation (PUI) for a high-risk pathogen, and specimens will be collected and handled following in-house protocols developed for a PUI in consideration of guidance from the Centers for Disease Control and Prevention (CDC). The periods of communicability (and the specimens at highest risk for transmission of infection in the laboratory) for various HHCDs warranting isolation (and potentially quarantine) are described in table 17.1.

Incubation periods differ among various diseases, but the contagious period for most pathogens generally begins after disease signs or symptoms are present. This principle is well established for the viral hemorrhagic fevers (VHFs). Influenza is a notable exception to this rule, and research has shown that influenza virus shedding and infectivity may occur 24 hours prior to the onset of symptoms. For other pathogens (SARS and MERS coronaviruses, for example) insufficient evidence is available to definitively establish the window of infectivity.

Specimens collected after the onset of signs and symptoms may carry a concentration of the pathogen that could result in infection of lab-oratorians from specimen collection, transport, analysis, and disposal. Exposure can occur through direct contact with mucus membranes, a sharps injury, or from inhaling an aerosol. Laboratorians should recognize, on a case-by-case basis, that certain specimens are riskier to handle than others. For example, respiratory specimens from an individual with a severe acute respiratory infection, such as coronavirus or avian influenza virus, will contain a higher concentration of virus than other body site specimens, whereas a patient infected with Ebola virus or Marburg virus may have extremely high concentrations in the blood, depending on the period of illness. Laboratorians, however, should recognize that any specimen could potentially contain a viable pathogen. For example, studies have identified virus in a variety of body fluids in patients with

Ebola virus disease, and virus shedding in stool was linked to clusters of SARS transmission during the 2003 outbreak.

Preanalytical Processes

As noted above, risk assessment for collection and transport of patient specimens is pathogen-specific. Specimens from asymptomatic persons in quarantine may be handled and analyzed in a manner identical to routine specimens, with the exception of novel influenza virus or other pathogens with potential for presymptomatic infectivity. Communication between the medical care team and laboratory personnel is essential during this observational period, as the situation could change rapidly and alter the risk dynamics. Assurances also need to be made to laboratory personnel that any specimen sent to the clinical laboratory will be appropriately labeled for tracking if an HHCD is subsequently identified. When a quarantined individual becomes symptomatic (now classified as a PUI), the laboratory protocol for collection and transport of specimens from this patient will need to be activated following communication between clinicians and the laboratory.

Laboratories are required to follow the appropriate local, state, or federal guidelines for specimen transport and surveillance reporting, which are dependent on the agent suspected. Facilities should plan and exercise collection and movement of specimens within the facility as well as packaging and shipping specimens for diagnostic testing outside of the facility, that is, to a Laboratory Response Network facility or to the CDC. All isolation unit and laboratory staff should be trained on US Occupational Safety and Health Administration (OSHA) Bloodborne Pathogens Standard (29 CFR 1910.1030), and personnel responsible for packaging and shipping potentially hazardous specimens should be proficient in US Department of Transportation Hazardous Materials Regulations (HMR) 49 CFR 171-180.

As a rule, specimens should be packaged for transport inside the isolation unit using redundant and shatterproof containment and surface decontamination, whether destined for the in-house laboratory or for an outside diagnostic facility. Procedures should minimize direct contact with specimen containers, facilitate rapid movement of specimens from isolation unit to destination, and minimize the number of people involved in the chain of movement. CDC guidelines for packaging and transport of a specimen that contains or may contain Ebola virus provide a reasonable general guide and can be accessed at https://www.cdc.gov/vhf/ebola/laboratory-personnel/specimens.html.

Analytical Processes

Safe handling and testing of specimens from a patient with the potential to have an HHCD in the clinical laboratory present particular laboratory biosafety challenges, and plans and procedures should be worked out in advance to enable safe operations and provide confidence for facility staff and the community at large. As with other activities in the isolation unit, the hierarchy of controls provides a framework for safe laboratory operations.

Ideally, facility plans can minimize or even eliminate the involvement of the main clinical laboratory in specimen processing and analysis. In many cases, point-of-care and small benchtop analyzers can facilitate bedside and satellite laboratory testing within the isolation unit itself, negating the need to move specimens outside of containment. In some cases, a small automated blood culture system within the isolation unit satellite lab are used.

In the event that bedside or in-unit laboratory testing is not feasible, utilization of the clinical laboratory should weigh the value of clinical laboratory information to be garnered from analysis with the risk presented to laboratory staff. Basic clinical laboratory testing, such as blood counts and chemistries, are critical in providing appropriate clinical care for patients with HHCDs, many of whom may be critically ill. The CDC's recommended test menu for the care of patients that are infected with Ebola virus can be accessed at https://www.cdc.gov/vhf/ebola/laboratory-personnel/safe-specimen-management.html.

Risk to staff can be mitigated through engineering and administrative controls that confine sample handling and testing to a remote or contained area of the laboratory with dedicated staff and equipment. If present, a clinical biosafety level 3 laboratory, such as a mycobacteriology or mycology laboratory section, provides preexisting controls that may be leveraged. Temporary containment structures that provide negative air pressure with HEPA-filtered exhaust can be purchased commercially. Specimens also could be processed and tested at off hours, allowing all unnecessary staff to vacate the lab and any cleaning or decontamination processes to occur prior to reinitiating normal laboratory shift work. Ideally, processing and testing should occur in automated and completely closed-loop analyzers and avoid procedures (such as centrifuging) with potential for aerosol generation. Laboratory staff should thoroughly investigate manufacturer guidance for the specific equipment located in the laboratory to understand any potential risk for aerosol generation and recommended decontamination procedures.

Finally, laboratory personnel handling HHCD specimens should wear appropriate personal protective equipment (PPE) for the specific pathogen in question. While some high-risk pathogens may present low epidemiological risk for aerosol transmission in the clinical setting (such as the filoviruses), certain laboratory procedures can create a higher chance for aerosolization. Aerosol protection with N-95 respirators or powered air-purifying respirators (PAPRs) is therefore generally recommended for laboratory staff working with specimens from a patient with an HHCD.

Postanalytical and Other Processes

Timely and accurate reporting of results closes the loop for clinical laboratory testing. To limit opportunities for communication breakdown, standard reporting processes should be used when possible. For security or other reasons, facilities may choose not to use standard health system inpatient or outpatient medical record systems for quarantined persons or patients in isolation. This situation will require precise communication between the medical care team and the laboratory, and alternate reporting systems should be planned and exercised in advance.

For clinical and public health applications, excess clinical material from specimens that have been collected from a person in isolation or quarantine should be appropriately stored if the need for additional testing is anticipated. Many high-risk pathogens are on the select agent list, and their handling is therefore subject to rules and regulations of the US Federal Select Agent Program (42 CFR Part 73). While clinical specimens are generally exempt from the requirements of select agent regulations, specimens from which a select agent has been confirmed are subject to these regulations 7 days after the conclusion of patient care. Any identification of a select agent from a clinical specimen should be reported to appropriate authorities immediately, and laboratory directors should contact the Division of Select Agents and Toxins at the CDC for specific guidance on handling these specimens. More information can be obtained at the program website: https://www.selectagents.gov /index.html.

Any laboratory supporting isolation and quarantine units should maintain a staff monitoring program to identify individuals who may have handled specimens from isolation patients or a quarantined individual, should this individual become ill from a high-risk pathogen. This will require that an occupational health program be implemented to allow monitoring of laboratorians and other individuals handling the specimens for the complete period of incubation (similar to what may be done for clinical providers exposed to patients with potentially hazardous infections), starting on the day with the last exposure to the specimen.

Finally, any HHCD that is thought to be from a potential deliberate exposure will be subject to investigation by appropriate law enforcement and counterterrorism authorities. In these cases, additional protocols for handling of specimens, such as maintenance of a chain-of-custody, may need to be implemented in conjunction with law enforcement protocols.

Conclusion

Laboratorians recognize the risks involved in handling human specimens on a routine basis. These personnel use appropriate PPE and follow the standard biosafety practices developed for the laboratory handling of specimens on a daily basis, which should facilitate planning for handling specimens from isolation or quarantine units. Nevertheless, high-risk pathogens present special challenges for laboratory operations, and a detailed plan and regular training will be critical in preventing laboratory-acquired infection. Communication between the medical care team and the clinical laboratory during periods of quarantine and, if applicable,

Table 17.1. Quarantinable Diseases and Their Periods of Contagion[a]

Disease(s)	Incubation period (days)[b]	Start of contagious period (days)[c]	Specimens of Highest Risk[d]
Influenza[e]	2–4	One day prior to symptoms	Respiratory secretions
Pneumonic plague	1–3	Onset of disease symptoms	Respiratory secretions
Monkeypox	7–17	Appearance of rash	Body fluids, lesions
MERS	2–14	Onset of disease symptoms	Respiratory secretions
SARS	2–14	Onset of disease symptoms	Respiratory secretions
Smallpox	10–14	Appearance of rash	Body fluids, lesions
Viral hemorrhagic fevers[f]	6–21	Onset of disease symptoms	Blood, other body fluids[g]

MERS = Middle Eastern respiratory syndrome; SARS = severe acute respiratory syndrome

[a]The contagious period and transmission routes for the various diseases are not always well defined and continue to raise uncertainties. Laboratory personnel use blood and body fluid precautions as a standard of practice.

[b]Time between exposure to a pathogen and symptom onset.

[c]When a person becomes contagious and most likely to transmit disease. Fever is the most common primary symptom recognized.

[d]Specimen(s) that are most likely to contain a concentration of the pathogen capable of transmitting disease in the laboratory.

[e]Includes any novel influenza virus that could cause a pandemic.

[f]Includes but not limited to South American hemorrhagic fevers, Crimean-Congo hemorrhagic fever, Ebola virus disease, Hendra virus disease, Lassa fever, Marburg hemorrhagic fever, Nipah virus encephalitis, and Rift Valley fever.

[g]Any specimen containing blood should be considered capable of transmitting disease in the laboratory, i.e., bloody sputum.

after the onset of signs and symptoms is a major component in the care of a quarantined individual or isolation patient. Regular interaction in planning and training will help provide for a safe environment for all individuals involved in the care of these unique cases.

CHAPTER 18

Transportation

JOCELYN J. HERSTEIN
KATELYN C. JELDEN
SHAWN G. GIBBS
MICHAEL L. FLUECKIGER
JOHN J. LOWE

The transport of patients harboring highly hazardous communicable diseases (HHCDs), as well those under investigation for high-risk exposures to these diseases, is a unique, challenging, and high-risk process. It is unlikely that a patient will initially present at a facility equipped with biocontainment and high-level containment care (HLCC) capabilities; instead, these patients are likely to require ground and/or air transport to a designated HLCC facility. Distinct from the stability of a clinical arena that offers advanced equipment, staffing teams, and specialized infrastructure, the transportation of patients infected with an HHCD in an aircraft or ground vehicle is conducted in a risky and fluctuating environment. A successful transport relies on extensive coordination and preplanning among a multitude of agencies (e.g., public health, law enforcement, transport agencies) and institutions (e.g., referring and receiving facilities); depending on the situation, participating groups can span local, state, federal, and international levels and may cross both geographical and political boundaries.

As an unpredictable environment, HHCD transport demands strict adherence to infection control principles, clear lines of communication, well-defined operational and tactical command, and the ability to adjust accordingly when necessary. Transportation of an HHCD patient should be well exercised, where possible, to ensure that proper protocols, procedures, and transportation routes are in place. Designated, trained transport teams with proven competence in infection control and patient loading and offloading procedures, as well as the necessary skill sets (e.g., medical, security, command, emergency response), increase the likelihood of a safe and successful transport and improve decision-making capacities during patient management en route. The appropriate selection and use of personal protective equipment (PPE) during the journey should be predetermined by expert risk assessment and thoroughly exercised. Waste disposal and vehicle decontamination following all phases of transport should be considered and discussed by appropriate parties. Monitoring of the patient transport team for signs of exposure and infection should be discussed in advance with the team; transport organization; and federal, state, and local health officials. A successfully executed HHCD patient transport will, of course, move the patient safely to their destination; however, it should also safeguard the workers conducting the transport, and in so doing safeguard the communities involved and minimize both the actual and perceived disruption to the public.

Ground Transport

Ground transport of patients with HHCDs requires highly detailed, planned protocols and involves coordination of multiple personnel and agencies. Procedures might encompass interfacility ground transport, airport-to-medical-facility transit, and movement from entry to patient placement within the medical facility. The entities involved in such transport might include the receiving medical facility, the referring medical facility, EMS services, aircraft transport teams, airport authorities, state and local health departments, state patrol and local police departments, the Federal Bureau of Investigation, the US State Department, county emergency management agencies, and the receiving medical facility's security team. Equipment will include appropriate PPE for transport personnel (e.g., powered air-purifying respirator [PAPR], Tychem® suit), individual patient isolation systems, communication devices (e.g., cell phones, radios), spill cleanup kits, and decontamination equipment.

Ground Transport Vehicles. A chase vehicle should follow the patient ambulance to coordinate communication between the ambulance and involved entities (e.g., police department, receiving medical facility) and provide supportive equipment and personnel as needed by the primary transport ambulance. For example, the chase vehicle might carry a spill cleanup kit, an individual patient isolation system, and duplicate PPE for staff within the ambulance as well as PPE for support personnel. Personnel in the chase vehicle might include an EMS captain, EMS physician, receiving medical facility staff, and referring medical facility staff. In some cases, a second ambulance may act as a chase vehicle to provide immediate redundancy if an issue arises with the primary transport ambulance.

Preparing the Ambulance. Personnel should consider preparing two ambulances for patient transport, one for primary transit and the other ready on standby. Of note, the use of a portable isolation system may negate the need for additional barrier protections to the ambulance. There are a variety of ways to prepare the ambulance; the authors have used the following process successfully. The patient compartment of the ambulance is draped ceiling to floor for barrier protection using one continuous piece of 6mm plastic sheeting, separating the driver compartment from the patient area. Every edge of the plastic sheeting should be sealed with duct tape, where the walls and ceiling meet and around the rear doors (figure 18.1). Lighting should not be covered, as it may heat the plastic and cause a fire hazard, and it may create a disorienting effect for the transport team. Medical equipment should be removed or stored in the patient compartment behind the plastic sheeting. A breach emergency box or other medical equipment needed for transport care should be stowed behind the plastic barrier in the patient compartment, cutting a flap in the plastic sheeting to allow access to stowed items but sealing the flap with duct tape until access is required. Ventilation in the driver's compartment should be operated for transport without use of recirculating air, while the exhaust vent in the patient compartment should be on. A disposable PPE barrier is placed on the stretcher. For the possibility of patient emesis, a bag for containment should be provided and the pillow and patient wrapped in an impermeable sheet to reduce contamination (e.g., an "adult transport cocoon" or "burrito wrap"). As an additional precaution, the patient may also be "self-contained" in PPE such as a Tychem® suit, procedure mask or N-95 respirator, gloves, and face shield; however, the patient must be able to tolerate these items. Given that the transport of a patient with an HHCD may garner media coverage, considerations should be made for covering the rear ambulance windows for patient privacy.

Interfacility Ground Transport Considerations. Local, state, and regional health departments cooperatively coordinate interfacility ground transport between receiving and referring medical facilities and EMS providers. Preparations for interfacility ground transport of patients with an HHCD must consider varying lengths in transport distance and time. The use of a chase vehicle/secondary ambulance might provide logistics support, health care personnel relief, assistance with refueling (if necessary), and emergency support. Paramedics and direct patient care staff should rotate out of direct patient care roles at least every 4 hours during transport. Long transports may require multiple EMS/ambulance teams with predetermined, safe patient transfer zones, designated PPE donning/doffing areas, and secure ambulance decontamination capacity. Locations for refueling, refueling procedures, and any potential jurisdictional issues should be addressed in advance of transport.

Medical Treatment Considerations. Care during transport of a patient with an HHCD must balance the benefits of treatment to a patient and the risks of contamination and infection to providers. Any altered standards of care should be outlined in advance with the transport organization's medical director, transport team, and referring and receiving physicians. A transfer consent form accompanies the patient from a referring facility and designates the receiving physician as the medical care provider. The referring and receiving physicians will direct treatment protocols and coordinate with the EMS medical director who guides EMS care during transport; the receiving physician should be immediately notified of any change in the patient's condition. Ideally, direct lines of communication should be established among the transport team, the EMS medical director, and the referring and receiving physicians. This will enable the

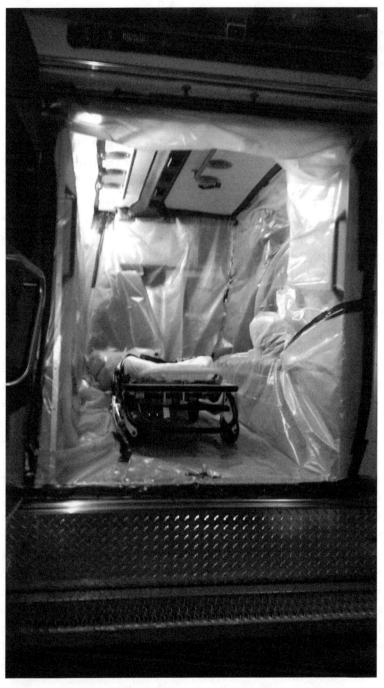

Figure 18.1. 6mm Plastic Sheeting Draping the Patient Compartment of an Ambulance with Duct Tape Sealing the Edges between Walls and Ceiling (Courtesy of UNMC)

provision of updates on medical status and guidance on care to be rendered by the transport team. Sharps use and invasive procedures should be minimized during transport and appropriate PPE worn by providers. If resuscitation is required, this should occur once the ambulance has stopped moving; however, it is also possible that compressions might be avoided during transport due to altered standards of care and patient acuity. Procedures should incorporate plans to safely contain bodily remains should a patient die during transit, likely continuing to the receiving facility where final remains processing could securely proceed.

Decontaminating the Ambulance. A location that is isolated, secure, and protected from the elements should be chosen for ambulance decontamination. Processes and plans for decontamination, packaging, and disposal of Category A waste and PPE, as well as facility security, should be established in advance. Although the authors successfully utilized the process presented, other decontamination processes are effective and may vary depending on causal pathogens. Personnel performing decontamination of the ambulance should wear appropriate PPE (e.g., full-face respirator with chemical and biological filters with Tychem® suit). Chemical and biological filters are recommended as ambulance space is confined and chemical fumes can accumulate quickly. Body fluid spills should first be contained, cleaned, and disinfected. While removing the 6mm plastic sheeting, sections should be rolled inward to prevent contamination of the outward ambulance surfaces and properly disposed of in biohazard bags. The plastic sheeting may need to be cut into smaller sections to safely fit inside biohazard bags or otherwise disposed of as Category A waste. If cutting of the plastic is necessary, trauma shears can be used to reduce the risk of injury to the worker. All surfaces within the ambulance should be cleaned with bleach wipes (or other Environmental Protection Agency [EPA]–approved disinfectant) twice, starting in "clean" areas (driver compartment) and finishing with "dirty" areas (patient compartment). A quality assurance observer should be present for decontamination to document the process and identify any breaches or potential contamination. Depending on the pathogen, a desiccation period may commence to allow organism inactivation. As a tertiary decontamination step, the patient compartment might be treated with ultraviolet germicidal irradiation or other gaseous (chlorine dioxide) or

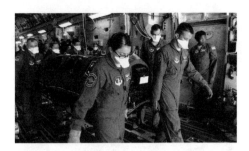

Figure 18.2. A Team Drills with the Air Force's Patient Isolation Unit (Courtesy of UNMC)

vaporous agents (hydrogen peroxide) that are EPA-approved for the causative agent.

Ground Transport Systems. Portable isolation systems contain a patient during ground transport and provide an extra layer of exposure protection for providers, particularly when used for very "wet" patients (i.e., patients with vomiting or diarrhea or otherwise emitting body fluids). However, as small and enclosed spaces, these systems are uncomfortable to the patient and limit direct patient care; as such, they may not be suitable for critically ill patients. In most HHCD cases, these portable isolators are single-use but may be reused if the disease is treatable and the unit can be decontaminated. The determination to reuse an isolator will be made in coordination with the local public health department and technical and clinical experts.

The ground transport systems described below are single-person isolation units that do not allow for direct patient care; rather, isolators are equipped with glove ports and sleeves for intravenous tubing for medical personnel external to the isolator to access the patient. Many of the commercially available patient isolation systems may be approved for ground transport but are not approved by the Federal Aviation Administration (FAA) for air transport. As large medical equipment will not fit into glove ports, it must be prepositioned within the isolator prior to patient placement. Each system is negatively pressurized and equipped with high-efficiency particulate air (HEPA) filtration.

The Patient Isolation Unit (PIU; figure 18.2) was first developed to protect US military service members from biological and chemical weapons in Iraq and Afghanistan. The single-occupancy, single-use containment unit is equipped with three HEPA filters that provide up to 12 air exchanges per hour. Exhaust ports are fitted with two chemical, biological, radiological, and nuclear (CBRN) filter cartridges. The base unit

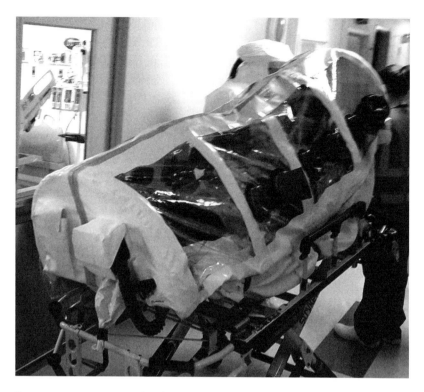

Figure 18.3. ISOPOD® Individual Patient Transport System (Courtesy of Nebraska Medicine)

enables interface with standard litter systems but includes 8 straps when litters are unavailable. Batteries enable the filter blowers to run for 16 hours, and a patient can be contained within the unit for up to 12 hours. The PIU was intended for use in both air and ground transportation.

The ISO-POD® (figure 18.3) is the brand name of an individual patient isolation system manufactured by Airboss of America Corporation. It is a lightweight, vinyl enclosure; the system and its components fit into a duffel bag and are assembled immediately prior to use. The ISO-POD® consists of two components: an isolation module and a filtration blower system capable of providing 21 air exchanges per hour. Restraint straps secure the patient during transport, and the durable, reinforced PVC lining is puncture resistant. ISO-POD® blowers run on a lithium ion battery that can provide up to 8 hours of operation; however, due to the small space and inability to control internal temperature, the ISO-POD® is unsuitable for lengthy transports. In recent years, several companies have produced different models of the individual patient isolation systems.

Route Selection. The selection of the most appropriate ground transport route is a decision based on extensive planning, coordination, and rehearsal. Selected and alternative transport routes should be preapproved by local and state authorities and the decision made in collaboration with local law enforcement, the state's transportation department, emergency management, and public health officials. Considerations for determining the most suitable route include jurisdictional authority and approval, the directness of the route to the receiving facility, the ability of road maintenance crews to respond to inclement weather, and traffic flow patterns. If applicable, the crossing of county and/or state borders should be minimized and routes selected so as to avoid entering governmental jurisdictions where the transport team does not have permission.

Local law enforcement agencies should be included in discussions on securing the selected route during transport, deciding if a law enforcement escort is needed, and responding to unanticipated problems or threats that may arise en route. Involvement of law enforcement agencies may also reduce transit times through traffic. During transport, predetermined communications methods (e.g., cell phones, secure radio channel) should be available to select participating agencies; these may include the receiving facility, transport team, law enforcement, and incident command.

Contingency plans should be thoroughly discussed prior to transport and should address issues that may arise en route; these may include vehicular accidents or failure, poor weather conditions, exposure of providers during transport, or breaches in PPE or isolator. Consider coordination with county emergency management during adverse weather to provide services such as snow plowing or road salting as necessary along the transport route.

Air Transport

The first documented aeromedical transportation of a patient infected with an HHCD was in 1970, when a patient infected with Lassa fever was transported from Nigeria to the United States for treatment. The patient was isolated in the first-class cabin of a scheduled Lufthansa flight without safety precautions for other passengers or crew; no secondary cases occurred. A second patient with Lassa fever was evacuated from Nigeria to Germany in 1974, utilizing barrier precautions and PPE. Around the same time, individualized patient isolators were developed to minimize transmission risks to evacuation staff. Over the last four decades, air transport technologies and systems have been developed to advance safety for transport teams while enabling access to the patient for en route care. During the 2014–16 outbreak of EVD in West Africa, at least 24 patients infected with EVD were transported to high-level isolation units in the United States and Europe with no secondary exposures en route.

Aeromedical transportation demands extensive coordination and collaboration. In the United States, the State Department is the coordinating agency for the transport of patients with confirmed or high-risk exposure to an HHCD from outside the continental United States, while the Department of Health and Human Services (HHS) is the coordinating agency for HHCD transports within the United States; other departments and agencies provide transport support. For transportation of a military service member, the Department of Defense (DoD) is the lead coordinating agency.

Aeromedical transport of patients infected with an HHCD can span lengthy time frames while adding stressors on the body, during which time patient status can significantly deteriorate and demand interventions that may heighten exposure risks to care providers and others on the aircraft. As such, systems have been developed with advanced capabilities to enable direct care of patients with an HHCD during an aeromedical evacuation while providing an environment that minimizes risks to health care professionals, other transport staff, and bystanders, and reduces the potential for aircraft contamination.

Air Transport Systems. Historically, individual containment systems were used to repatriate patients infected with HHCDs. Despite confined patient space and limited patient care capabilities, individual isolators, such as the PIU and air transport isolator (ATI; figure 18.4), have been used for decades and could be employed for both air and ground trans-

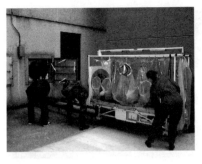

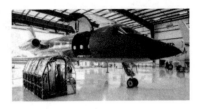

Figure 18.5 The ABCS with Its
Transport Aircraft (Photo by
CDC)

Figure 18.4. A Team from USAMRIID
Prepares to Move a Patient in the Air
Transport Isolator (Photo by
USAMRIID)

port. During the 2014–16 EVD outbreak, the system used for the majority of aeromedical evacuations of infected patients, known as the aeromedical biological containment system (ABCS; figure 18.5), allowed for direct patient care; however, it too was a single-patient system.

Limitations to a single-person system exist. A single transport capability requires prioritization of patient acuity, increased expenses, and potential delays in treatment of a second patient due to time needed to conduct the first transport, as well as the need to decontaminate the aircraft, reset staff, and return to impacted areas. These limitations have since led to the development of systems capable of transporting multiple patients. In most cases, these devices will need FAA approval to be utilized on an aircraft. However, use on military aircraft or outside of the United States may have different standards for which devices are considered safe to fly.

The British Royal Air Force (RAF) developed the ATI in the 1970s, and a similar system (Vickers Air Transport Isolator [VATI]) was used by the US military for several decades. Prior to the 2014–16 outbreak of EVD, the RAF maintained three isolators that were used on four occasions; however, a reassessment during the EVD outbreak led to the development of an additional 25 ATIs. In 2014, the RAF transported a patient infected with EVD from West Africa to Britain in the ATI. Smaller than the units detailed below, the ATI and VATI can be used for both in-flight and ground transport: the isolator can be transferred from the aircraft to an awaiting ground vehicle and transported to the treatment facility with the patient only leaving the isolator on admission into the containment unit. A negative pressure unit equipped with HEPA filtration, the system includes an intubation suit with gloves and a face shield to allow greater airway support, and ports

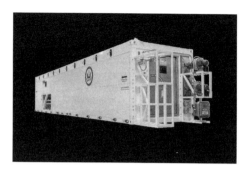

Figure 18.6 The CBCS (Courtesy of MRIGlobal under Contract to DoS)

enable equipment and drugs to be passed into the isolator. A tube extension at the foot of the unit allows clinical waste to be isolated from the patient during transport.

The ABCS was developed through a cooperative agreement between the Centers for Disease Control and Prevention (CDC), DoD, and Phoenix Air Group (PAG). First operationalized in 2007, the system had not been used until the 2014–16 outbreak in West Africa, during which the system was employed by PAG for the aeromedical transport of 41 patients, including 24 to high-level isolation units in the United States and Europe. Designed to prevent the escape of airborne pathogens, the ABCS consists of an anteroom and a patient chamber with negative pressure and a redundant HEPA-filtered ventilation system. A metal frame supports a clear polyvinyl chloride liner that enables medical professionals to provide direct care to the patient inside the unit. The ABCS is designed for the transport of a single patient; following patient transport, the system is disassembled and the liner, waste, and HEPA filters sent to an incinerator via a licensed Category A waste vendor.

In 2015, to address the limitation of a single-patient transport system, the US Department of State partnered with the Paul G. Allen Foundation in a public-private partnership with MRIGlobal to develop, fabricate, and certify a next-generation HHCD transport system with the capability of moving multiple patients in a single system. As of 2018, two containerized biological containment systems (CBCSs, figure 18.6)

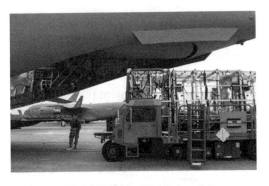

Figure 18.7 The TIS Being Loaded onto Its Transport Aircraft (Photo by USAF)

have been constructed; both are owned and operated by the US State Department and maintained by PAG. The CBCS consists of a medical staff room, an anteroom, and a patient treatment room with area to provide critical care for up to 4 patients for 16 hours. The system is equipped with negative pressure, HEPA filtration, and video monitoring. Built within a 40-foot shipping container, the hard, rigid surfaces of the CBCS facilitate ease of decontamination using combined quaternary ammonium disinfectant and vaporous hydrogen peroxide.

In 2014, the DoD contracted Productions Product to develop a system that provided multipatient isolation capabilities for service members who may have had a high-risk exposure to EVD. A modular, expandable system, the Transport Isolation System (TIS, figure 18.7) includes an anteroom and one or more patient care modules equipped with negative pressure, HEPA filtration, and watertight enclosures to protect the aircraft and exterior crew. TIS modules utilize the Standard Patient Support Pallet system, allowing for adjustable configuration of seats and litters. Multiple ports for oxygen tubing, monitoring cables, and electric cords allow for large medical equipment and devices to be placed external to the TIS while maintaining the ability for aeromedical evacuation crews and critical care teams to provide direct patient care. Production Products manufactured 25 TISs in 2015; the systems are positioned in 4 bases across the contiguous United States.

Air Transport Platforms. There are a variety of both fixed-wing and rotary aircraft that can be utilized to transport patients with HHCDs; the selection of aircraft will depend on factors that include availability, aircraft range, and the capability to hold the air transportation systems and associated support equipment and staff. Smaller fixed-wing aircraft and rotary aircraft can be used to move the individual patient isolators (e.g., PIU and ATI), as was the case in 2014 when both an unspecified helicopter and a Cessna 208 transported patients with EVD within Guinea one at a time in an individual patient isolation system they referred to as a Human Stretcher Transit Isolation-total Containment (Oxford) Limited. PAG has utilized a modified Gulfstream G3 for transportation of patients within their ABCS intercontinentally and within the United States and Europe. The DoS's CBCS can be moved within a Boeing 747 aircraft, drastically increasing the flight range to 7,260 nautical miles and thus allowing for intercontinental transports without the need for a refueling stop. The TIS has been approved for use on the USAF C17 Globemaster III and the USAF C-130, which have an unrefueled range of 2,400 and 1,800 nautical miles, respectively; however, both systems have midair refueling capabilities and therefore an almost unlimited range. The C-130 requires a smaller takeoff and landing distance and thus can use smaller and less robust airfields than both the C17 and 747, providing accessibility to more remote locations.

The geopolitical aspects regarding the flight path and refueling stops must be addressed in advance with a number of parties, including the CDC, DoS, and FAA. For example, the modified Gulfstream G3 air ambulance operated by PAG during the 2014 EVD outbreak required two stops for refueling and had to pass through US Customs Service during its trip from West Africa to the continental United States, both of which needed permission from the appropriate national authorities. These landings had to be delicately coordinated in advance to minimize the actual and political disruption to the airports and communities in which they are situated. Some countries (or even US states) could potentially refuse to permit the landing of aircraft with HHCD patients onboard.

If there is a need to decontaminate any portion of the aircraft, only methods (chemical and physical) approved by the FAA and the aircraft manufacturer should be used to ensure aircraft airworthiness is not compromised. For example, many chemical disinfectants may deteriorate seals and other components of an aircraft that help maintain its pressurization, which could lead to catastrophic failure.

Air-to-Ground Handoff. The handoff of a patient from an arriving aircraft to an awaiting ground transport team requires extensive preplanning and communication. Identifying the location of patient transition is important to reduce handoff time, minimize environmental exposure, and conceal the process from media and bystanders both for their safety and for the privacy of the patient. All involved parties should be updated on clinical status during the air transport to aid in ground crew preparation and expectations (e.g., transport of ambulatory or litter patient). On arrival, a team lead from the air evacuation team should brief awaiting ground transport crews on patient status and changes that may have occurred in-flight. Patients should be offloaded in protective PPE or in an isolator, as indicated. Ground transport teams should notify the receiving facility of patient status and estimated time of arrival.

Movement of the PUI to Isolation

A person or patient under investigation (PUI) is an individual who is both symptomatic and has had exposure to an HHCD. The PUI has not been confirmed as having the disease in question through laboratory testing, but an HHCD is suspected and has not been ruled out. Another individual category of concern is a person who has had a high-risk exposure (HRE) to an HHCD (i.e., needlestick or contaminated fluid splash to the eyes), but is not currently exhibiting symptoms. Both the PUI and the person with an HRE require extensive coordination among public health officials and clinicians to determine the best course of action for both the PUI/HRE and the potentially impacted communities. Transporting a PUI or person with an HRE to a location in close proximity of an HLCC facility may be preferable in certain situations; for example, when the PUI or person with an HRE is early in the disease course or asymptomatic and are located in an environment with insufficient resources to provide effective care on escalated symptoms and confirmed disease. If a PUI or individual with an HRE is a health care provider responding to an outbreak, movement may also be sought; treatment of a known colleague could be detrimental to the morale of health care workers (many of whom are likely to be volunteers) and subsequently the overall mission.

Despite a lack of laboratory confirmation, PUI movement should proceed as though the PUI were a confirmed patient in order to protect transport teams and communities involved. If disease was later confirmed, no additional exposures should have arisen from the transport process. Similar to a confirmed case, the suspected disease and the transmissibility of the causal pathogen will drive the level of precautions, such as PPE and engineering controls.

Waste infected with certain highly hazardous pathogens must be transported and disposed of as Category A waste according to the US Department of Transportation (DOT). The waste produced during transport of a PUI will likely be considered Category A waste (such was the case with EVD); therefore, it should be handled and packaged as such, following DOT and other applicable state and local regulations. If an HHCD is later ruled out, state and local government regulations would determine whether the associated patient waste would still be handled as Category A waste or if it could be disposed of as Category B medical waste.

The transport of an individual with an HRE, in contrast, may allow for some flexibility in the amount and types of controls utilized. By definition, these persons are asymptomatic. If the disease is only transmitted while symptomatic, as is the case with the vast majority of infectious diseases, the individual might be transported with less stringent precautions; however, a contingency plan should be available if symptoms develop. For example, numerous individuals with HREs to EVD were transported in a private aircraft with isolation capabilities. Although these individuals remained outside the isolation unit, the contingency plan involved their movement into the onboard unit if they became symptomatic. Moreover, if transport is conducted within the established incubation period for a known causal pathogen, additional precautions may be unnecessary. For example, the known incubation period for Lassa virus is 6 to 21 days. If an individual were exposed via needlestick and was rapidly transported by ambulance to a facility within hours, the transit may be completed with little or no controls as it would be completed well before the established incubation period; again, contingency plans should still be in place. Depending on state and local regulations, waste generated by an HRE may not require special disposal methodologies.

Intramural Transport

Transport of a patient with an HHCD from the entrance of a medical facility into an HLCC unit necessitates prioritization of the safety of those within the medical facility, emphasizing security, decontamination procedures, and rapid patient movement. Intramural routes should utilize direct pathways while minimizing environmental exposure risks. If ambulatory, the patient may walk or be moved by wheelchair into the isolation unit via the most direct route. The receiving medical facility should assemble a receiving team composed of isolation unit staff experienced in decontamination procedures. Wearing appropriate PPE based on patient acuity and containment, the transport team escorts the patient from facility entry until isolation unit placement. Facility security restricts all public access to the patient transport route until decontamination is complete and should be positioned greater than 15 feet from the patient route at all times; security is instructed not to approach the patient and transport team but to keep the public away. The receiving team should clean spills immediately with prepared spill kits (e.g., bleach wipes, mop and bucket, absorbent wipes). After the patient is placed in the isolation unit, the receiving team performs a full decontamination of the transport route within the medical facility, from the patient entry point to within the isolation unit.

Conclusion

Extensive planning and exercising of transportation procedures ensures that comprehensive procedures exist and communication structures for numerous agencies have been tested.

Isolation systems developed for aeromedical and ground transport minimize secondary transmission risks to transport teams. Single-use, individual patient isolators for ground transportation encase a patient in a negative-pressure environment while glove ports enable access for patient care. The development of larger, multipatient transport systems for aeromedical isolation provide biocontainment-level infrastructure, enable direct care, and expand the capacity of transports to four or more suspected or confirmed HHCD patients. However, few such systems are currently available. While the EVD outbreak in 2014–16 resulted in relatively few international evacuations that were within the means of one organization, a larger outbreak requiring aeromedical evacuation of more patients would demand greater global capacity.

Although significant developments have been made in transportation capabilities since the 2014–16 outbreak of EVD, the transportation of patients with HHCDs is underexplored. Research and development into this area is needed to advance methods and systems to protect transport teams while supporting sophisticated patient care.

CHAPTER 19

Waste Handling

CHRISTOPHER K. BROWN*
AURORA B. LE
SELIN B. HOBOY
SHAWN G. GIBBS

Introduction

The 2014–16 West Africa Ebola epidemic and treatment of 11 patients in the United States presented unique logistical challenges to federal, state, and local entities not encountered routinely. Handling of infectious wastes from the patients was no exception. The waste generated by the patients, both solid and liquid, was not the only aspect requiring attention. The proper disposal of personal protective equipment (PPE) worn by health care providers, bed linens, items used to decontaminate medical equipment and surfaces in the room, and any other objects that came into contact with the patients during transport and treatment needed to be disposed of properly as a critical step of infection control due to potential or actual pathogen contamination. Even materials that infected individuals came into contact with in their homes or in public spaces had to be managed appropriately.

Waste contaminated with—or suspected to be contaminated with—Ebola virus and other pathogens capable of causing highly hazardous communicable diseases (HHCDs) can be inactivated effectively utilizing existing decontamination or sterilization methods, including incinera-

---

* This work was written in the author's personal capacity and does not necessarily represent the views of the US Department of Labor/Occupational Safety and Health Administration.

tion and autoclaving. Once infectious waste has been appropriately incinerated, autoclaved, or otherwise inactivated by a validated process in order to eliminate the specific pathogen, it is no longer considered a hazardous material under federal law. Ideally, such waste should be properly inactivated at the site where it was generated; however, over the past several decades, many health care facilities have decommissioned their on-site incinerators, and few have sufficient autoclave capacity to support treating the large volume of waste associated with HHCD patient care. The alternative, transporting infectious waste for treatment at off-site facilities, is potentially more hazardous to workers, more complex from a compliance perspective, and tends to draw greater public scrutiny. Any US medical facility providing care for patients with HHCDs but lacking the ability to inactivate the waste on-site needs to ensure that its personnel are trained to properly and safely package the waste, procure proper packaging materials for transport, and work with a medical waste transporter that has the appropriate qualifications, including all potentially applicable state permits, a US Department of Transportation (DOT) special permit, proper insurance, and so on. Facilities need to ensure that the waste they are releasing will be disposed of at a properly permitted treatment facility. This chapter details the complexities of managing HHCD or Category A infectious wastes throughout the waste life cycle, from generation through on-site treatment, packaging, transportation, and off-site treatment to ultimate disposal. It also examines associated risks, as well as considerations and suggestions for both solid and liquid waste management.

Waste Regulations

Management of waste associated with isolation and quarantine must be done in a manner that complies with a complex framework of requirements at the federal, state or territorial, and, in some cases, local levels. Laws, regulations, and local ordinances (if applicable) may apply differently to solid and liquid waste, as well as to different categories of potentially hazardous or infectious waste. This section discusses some of the most important examples.

Several federal agencies regulate potentially infectious waste at various stages of its life cycle. Perhaps most pertinent for solid waste are the Hazardous Materials Regulations (HMR; 49 Code of Federal Regulations [CFR] Parts 171–180) of the DOT. The HMR cover the transportation of all hazardous materials, including those contaminated with or otherwise containing material designated as Category A and Category B infectious substances. The most virulent organisms, including Ebola viruses, which are present in a form capable of causing permanent disability or life-threatening disease in otherwise healthy humans or animals, comprise Category A, while those that are not life-threatening, fatal, or disability-inducing, including those found in waste generated through routine patient care, make up Category B. Importantly, specimens potentially containing certain organisms, such as Ebola and some other hemorrhagic fever viruses, are always considered Category A, while others, such as *Bacillus anthracis*, are considered Category A only when they are intentionally propagated (i.e., cultured). Regulated medical wastes, which include waste or reusable material derived from the medical treatment of an animal or human, that contain an infectious substance must be classified as either Category A or Category B, depending on the substance(s) known or suspected to be in the waste and the form that these substances are in (e.g., cultures versus patient waste only). Category A waste, which is assigned United Nations (UN) identification numbers 2814 (infectious substances, affecting humans) or 2900 (infectious substances, affecting animals), must be managed according to the HMR's packaging, marking, and shipping requirements for Category A infectious substances when transported in commerce (i.e., by commercial waste haulers) via air, highway, rail, or water. When Category B materials (designated UN 3373) become waste, they are then assigned identification number UN 3291 and have their own specific set of packaging requirements.

The categorical designations applied to potentially infectious solid waste under the HMR are independent of the classification of waste as hazardous under Environmental Protection Agency (EPA) requirements and the authority of the Resource Conservation and Recovery Act

(RCRA). Generally, the HMR govern the methods by which hazardous materials or hazardous waste is moved between locations, while RCRA regulations set requirements as to how hazardous waste must be managed at landfills and other hazardous waste treatment facilities. RCRA requirements specify measures for protecting the environment from hazardous materials that could leach out of landfills if they are not properly contained, especially those that may persist in the environment, bioaccumulate, or otherwise have a lasting negative environmental impact.

Many activities that generate potentially infectious waste or involve workers managing such waste also trigger worker protection requirements enforced by the Occupational Safety and Health Administration (OSHA), such as the agency's Bloodborne Pathogens (29 CFR 1910.1030) and PPE (29 CFR 1910 Subpart I) standards. Some states that operate their own OSHA-approved safety and health programs also have similar, if not more stringent, worker health and safety requirements. Generally, these requirements obligate employers to assess hazards that could lead to worker exposures, identify ways to reduce or eliminate those hazards in order to protect workers, and train workers to perform their jobs safely. Depending on the circumstances, state and federal occupational safety and health requirements apply throughout much of the typical waste life cycle.

STATE REQUIREMENTS

Most states set their own requirements for the management and treatment of infectious medical wastes. This state-by-state approach leads to significant variability among states. Some states regulate medical waste as part of a broad set of requirements for all solid waste, often under the authority of their environmental protection agencies. Other states use a combination of solid waste regulations and health department requirements—and these regulatory measures may not always fully align, especially when it comes to managing highly infectious waste. Some states also require various types of regulated medical waste to be managed in a specific way, while others allow some or all regulated medical waste to be put directly into specialized or appropriately permitted landfills. In many cases, states that require treatment allow for either incineration through a permitted hospital medical infectious waste incinerator (HMIWI) or autoclaving with a properly validated process. Alternative treatment technologies may be permitted but must often go through additional validation processes.

These state-by-state differences, as well as intrastate differences among various environmental and health departments, created considerable challenges during the management of Ebola-contaminated Category A waste. Few, if any, states were prepared to deal with Category A waste (other than routine research laboratory specimens) and the potential hazards, both real and perceived, associated with managing this type of waste stream. Some states took extreme measures, prohibiting waste haulers from moving such materials through their state or requiring a police escort to do so. More measured approaches required waste treatment facilities accepting material from health care institutions to validate microbial inactivation protocols ahead of waste acceptance.

Management of Solid Waste

Waste contaminated with—or suspected to be contaminated with—pathogens capable of causing HHCDs, including Ebola virus, can be managed safely and effectively. However, doing so requires careful planning, in advance of patient admission, which considers the complete waste life cycle and applicable federal, state or territorial, and local requirements. Facilities that might accept patients with HHCDs, whether to triage, stabilize, and transfer them to better-equipped hospitals, or to treat them as patients in their own specialized biocontainment units, should work with local and state health and environmental departments to understand their requirements. Additionally, facilities should discuss capabilities and options with their contracted waste management companies to ensure all involved are aware of and in agreement with a waste management plan in advance of accepting a patient or a potential outbreak.

Several considerations related to waste generation in quarantine and isolation settings can simplify downstream waste management steps. Minimizing the total amount of waste generated by taking only necessary supplies into patient care or other contaminated areas is a best practice. When waste is generated, it should be segregated into Category A regulated medical waste, Category B regulated medical waste, or waste that may be disposed of in standard municipal trash streams. This can potentially reduce the amount of bona fide Category A waste and alleviate challenges associated with on- and off-site storage, treatment, and disposal of unnecessarily large amounts of materials.

When waste is generated, it should be stored in a secure area accessible only to appropriately trained and protected essential personnel. Facilities should consider the rate of anticipated waste generation, as well as their capacity to treat that waste or the frequency with which a waste hauler will collect it, when determining where and how to store the waste. Care of patients with severe disease, especially those with viral hemorrhagic fevers who produce copious amounts of feces and vomitus, as well as items contaminated with blood and other body fluids, may generate eight to ten 55-gallon drums of used PPE, medical supplies, linens, and other material waste per day. Although it may vary based on the duration an ill patient is hospitalized, along with other factors, total waste from a single Ebola patient over the course of hospitalization has been shown to exceed sixty (60) 55-gallon drums.

Some health care facilities may plan to treat solid waste on-site through a variety of means. One such method is autoclaving, a steam sterilization process in which heat is applied to the waste in a highly pressurized chamber for a specified time and at a specified temperature and pressure in order to render pathogens nonviable. Most pathogens can be inactivated using a facility's on-site autoclave capabilities, but waste management contracts may also augment this capability with portable autoclaves. In either case, treating waste with a validated autoclave cycle, typically heating for a minimum of 30 minutes at 250°F, ensures it is no longer infectious. Standard procedure involves the use of spores as biological indicators of the autoclave's ability to inactivate organisms. Autoclaving processes are typically validated to reduce viable organisms by 10^{-4} or 10^{-6}—for example, a reduction of 1 million organisms to either 100 or 1, respectively. This validation should be done with sample waste or dunnage similar to the wastes the facility anticipates accepting for treatment, prior to using the autoclave for actual infectious waste. This is important to ensure that treatment protocols effectively inactivate waste with viable pathogens. After validation and during the course of treating waste, spore testing and parametric monitoring can ensure that autoclave cycles achieve appropriate time and temperature to inactivate pathogens in the waste.

Incinerating waste, especially bulkier items such as mattresses and draperies, can achieve similar results by reducing the material to ashes. Once Ebola-associated waste has been appropriately incinerated, autoclaved, or inactivated by another validated means, it is no longer deemed hazardous material under federal law since pathogens in the material have been inactivated. However, as previously noted, the chief stipulation at the time of the 2014–16 outbreak was that, in the United States, the Ebola-associated waste needed to be properly inactivated on-site.

Without on-site autoclave or incineration capabilities, facilities generating infectious waste need to plan to transport the waste for off-site treatment. This waste material must be packaged according to applicable DOT HMR requirements, which are more stringent for Category A waste than for Category B or regular regulated medical waste. For all waste to which the HMR apply, containers must be leak-proof, properly marked, and accompanied by hazardous materials shipping papers. Category A infectious substances require more complex and protective packaging to ensure that waste materials are safe for transport.

Prior to the 2014–16 Ebola outbreak, there were no standard packaging options for waste larger than typical laboratory samples. DOT had to issue a special permit and instructions to allow for packaging accommodations so that waste haulers could transport waste materials from health care facilities to a treatment facility.

When infectious waste is packaged appropriately, it is usually not necessary to pretreat the waste with a disinfectant prior to moving it off-site for treatment. Disinfectant added to waste is usually unable to penetrate porous materials, so the waste remains potentially infectious. However, moving waste that has not yet been autoclaved or incinerated likely means that downstream treatment and disposal workers will need additional protections compared to workers managing only autoclave residuals. This is also why it is critical for health care staff packaging the waste be properly trained on all packaging and closure protocols.

Although this chapter is not intended to address off-site treatment and disposal, note that these stages of the waste life cycle should be considered as part of any waste management plan. Entities that anticipate generating waste themselves or managing waste generated elsewhere, including in infected individuals' homes, should consider the ultimate destination of such waste if it is not fully inactivated on site, how it will get there, and where the final product—including autoclave residual or incinerator ash—will be sent.

Management of Liquid Waste and Effluents

There remains limited scientific information regarding the survivability and health hazards within wastewater associated with organisms that cause HHCDs. Emerging studies demonstrate that the Ebola virus can survive in US wastewater for days, posing a potential health hazard to wastewater workers, but that the Ebola virus in wastewater is susceptible to sodium hypochlorite—a commonly used disinfectant.

Multiple federal laws and regulations focus on overall water quality and source water protection, but they do not provide definitive advice regarding liquid waste and effluents from suspected or confirmed HHCD patients in isolation and quarantine. CDC guidance allowing for the untreated release of liquid waste from confirmed patients with Ebola virus disease would also apply to those under quarantine or isolation for unconfirmed Ebola and certain other HHCDs. However, it is important to consult state and local laws and regulations when planning for the management of liquid waste and effluents from those within isolation and quarantine. If no state and local laws and regulations governing the discharge of these types of wastes can be found, it is recommended that discussion of these scenarios and procedures with state and local officials be conducted, including those from the local municipal wastewater treatment plant (WWTP) or publicly owned treatment works (POTW).

Biosafety level 3 and 4 (BSL-3 and 4) laboratories, under the Federal Select Agent Program, are required to pretreat their liquid waste prior to discharge into the WWTP, and the US Army Medical Research Institute of Infectious Diseases (USAMRIID) chemically pretreats its liquid waste and also steam-sterilizes it prior to discharge. Existing biocontainment units in the United States that have treated patients known or suspected to have Ebola virus disease also opted to chemically pretreat liquid waste prior to discharge. Given the many unanswered questions, and the current precedence set by BSL-3 and 4 laboratories, as well as biocontainment units, isolation and quarantine facilities should develop their own standard operating procedure (SOP) for the pretreatment of liquid waste and effluent prior to WWTP/POTW discharge.

Protecting Workers during Waste Management Activities

A critical consideration in planning for both solid and liquid waste management is protecting worker health and safety. There are numerous opportunities for worker exposure to potentially infectious waste or contaminated materials. These may occur at various points throughout the waste life cycle, including, but not limited to, situations wherein workers are collecting, packaging, moving, opening, or otherwise coming in contact with waste or waste containers. In solid waste streams in particular, sharp objects, such as needles, scalpels, and broken glass, can cause puncture wounds, cuts, and other percutaneous injuries that can lead to worker infections. Workers may also be exposed to chemicals when pretreating solid or liquid waste.

As in the case of other occupational health hazards, it is necessary for health care, waste management, and other employers to perform a thorough hazard assessment to identify if, how, when, and where their workers may be at risk of exposure to potentially infectious materials, dangerous chemicals, or other hazards. Following the hierarchy of controls (see chapter 8) consistently applied to workplace health and safety hazards, employers can then determine what types of engineering controls, administrative controls, safe work practices, and PPE should be used to protect workers. Existing OSHA standards for bloodborne pathogens (29 CFR 1910.1030) and PPE (29 CFR 1910 Subpart I) may require employers to provide certain types of controls, as well as worker training, medical exams, and other measures that, together, are part of a comprehensive protection program for waste workers or others with waste management duties.

Conclusion

The 2014–16 West Africa Ebola outbreak and the subsequent treatment of patients in the United States required health care and affiliated sectors to work through the logistics of Category A waste management and transport on a large scale, for the first time. The handling of waste is a challenging and critical component of isolation and quarantine care. As such, the importance of planning for, and coordination of, such handling prior to patient acceptance cannot be overstated.

Ongoing work aims to create standards and guidance for the next HHCD event. Nevertheless, effective HHCD waste management that ensures the safety of all workers involved requires clearly delineated SOPs that take into account contingencies, appropriate acquisition of permits and packaging materials—or at least a relationship with a supplier from which those materials could be readily obtained—and coordination, partnership, and trust with affiliated federal, state, and local stakeholders will be pivotal in future scenarios. Especially in a world of emerging and reemerging HHCDs, it is only a matter of time before health care facilities and related organizations face the complexities of managing highly infectious waste again—ideally with better preparation the next time.

CHAPTER 20

Care of the Deceased

KATE C. BOULTER

ANGELA M. VASA

When providing care to patients infected with a highly hazardous communicable disease (HHCD), everyone's goal is to optimize their chances to survive and discharge them to live a long and happy life, but an unfortunate reality is that patients may not survive. Because death is an inevitable part of life, there are many traditions and rituals that have developed around when someone passes such as washing the body, touching a loved one, dressing them in their favorite clothes, and many more. Depending on the HHCD, none of these may be possible, and in some cases, families may not have a choice regarding the final disposition. If burial is the desired option and allowable by public health entities, there may be specific accommodations required. The casket may need to be sealed and the body contained in several layers of mortuary bags due to the postmortem viability of the pathogen. In other situations, such as the presence of an implanted pacemaker in the decedent that won't be removed, cremation may be excluded as temperatures as high as 2400°F may cause the lithium battery to explode inside the cremator.

This chapter will focus on procedures that should be followed in a setting such as the United States. Significant human-to-human spread of viral hemorrhagic fever (most from Ebola viruses) has occurred in African settings related to contacts with the deceased during outbreaks. Much experience has been gained in those settings by working with communities to conduct safe, dignified burials that attempt to incorporate families and communities in the preparation and interment process.

There is a fine balance between respecting the decedent's cultural traditions and ensuring the health and safety of those who come in contact with the body. For the health care provider, there are many facets to providing postmortem care for a deceased patient, but the most critical is the need to understand the risk of disease transmission after death. Understanding the hazards and postmortem stability of an organism will inform the provider on the appropriate infection control measures that need to be in place to protect those who are preparing the body and prevent the spread of infection in the community at large. The Ebola virus is an example of a pathogen capable of postmortem transmission as it remains viable for up to 7 days on the skin, and longer in blood and body cavities. The ability of the Ebola virus to spread postmortem resulted in many second- and third-generation infections during the 2014–16 West Africa Ebola outbreak, as was demonstrated in a case study where 28 individuals who participated in the burial practices of just one decedent contracted the disease. In addition to knowing how to protect oneself, it is essential to be knowledgeable of the law regulating mortuary affairs.

Legal and Policy Considerations

Legal and policy considerations have two main points of focus: the health and safety of workers and the issues related to the containment and final disposition of the remains. Workers are protected by the Occupational Safety and Health Act of 1970, which requires employers to provide employees with a workplace that is free from recognized hazards that are capable of causing severe physical harm or death. However, when the hazard is unavoidable, as in the case of providing postmortem care for a body infected with the Ebola virus, the General Duty Clause Section 5(a)(1) requires employers to take reasonable measures to lessen the risk from hazards. These measures can include the provision of personal protective equipment (PPE) and the development of protocols and training programs to direct safe practices. Additionally, employers must comply with the Bloodborne Pathogens standard (29 CFR 1910.1030) if there is a potential for the employee to come in contact with blood or other potentially infectious materials. This includes the provision of tools and devices engineered for safety, employee postexposure contingency plans, and annual training, regardless of the employees' past training and education. Federal guidelines on the containment of infected human remains are provided by the Centers for Disease Control and Prevention (CDC), but laws that govern the disposition of the deceased are provided by individual state statutes. Each state has its own regulations that govern the transportation and disposition of human remains. Generally, if it is determined that a hazard exists that could cause harm to a community, state governors can issue public health orders to direct measures to mitigate the risk. This may include a mandate for cremation instead of burial, but each state is unique in this regard.

Preparing and Containing the HHCD-infected Human Remains

The manner in which HHCD-infected human remains are prepared for cremation or interment will largely depend on guidance provided by the World Health Organization (WHO), the CDC, and each state's public health department (PHD). In some cases, it is possible that normal processes will be sufficient, or it may be judicious to place a surgical mask over the decedent's airway if there is concern for pathogens being forced out of the mouth or nose during manipulation of the decedent. Another method to consider is to wrap the decedent in fluid-impermeable material prior to placement in a mortuary bag if there is concern for pathogens that transmit by contact. It is not unreasonable to anticipate that if the disease process and treatment activities of a patient result in waste generation classified as Category A hazardous material (see chapter 19), the CDC or PHD may issue guidelines that reflect what was advised during the 2014–16 West Africa Ebola outbreak. In that situation, the CDC provided guidance for the safe handling of human remains infected with Ebola virus disease for US health care facilities and mortuaries, which includes a detailed process for postmortem preparation, transportation, and disposition of the remains. The instructions emphasize Ebola's propensity for postmortem transmission, and accentuate the notion that only trained personnel should handle Ebola-infected human remains. Training should include instruction on how to use the equipment while wearing PPE. Practices normally associated with postmortem care of a patient, including bathing the body and removing medical equipment such as intravenous lines, endotracheal tubes, and pacemakers, is not advised. Embalmment and autopsy are also contraindicated; exceptions should only occur under guidance of the CDC. Burial is permitted but ultimately is at the discretion of individual state health departments. Some states have mandated cremation for Ebola-infected remains.

Preparing the decedent for transportation is a 21-step process designed to secure the remains within three different grades of mortuary bags. The process requires sectioning the working area into hot and cold zones with two distinct teams in each zone. The hot zone will require at least four personnel, while the cold zone can be managed with a team of two. The entire process requires strict infection control procedures with staff adhering meticulously to protocol to minimize the risk of cross contamination between the two teams. The hot zone team prepares and contains the body within three mortuary bags, while the cold zone team avoids any contact with the remains and any potentially contaminated surfaces. The role of the team in the cold zone is to receive the contained remains and proceed with transportation.

Required equipment (which must be moved into the patient's room [i.e., the hot zone]) includes:

- A hospital gurney.

- 3 mortuary bags opened and positioned on the gurney in the reverse order in which they will be used:
  - The outermost layer and third bag to be used (which should be placed on the bottom) is an 18-mil thickness (457 micrometers) heavy-duty mortuary bag made from laminated vinyl or compatible chlorine-free material that will contain the remains after they have been sealed within the heat-sealed pouch. Other specifics of this bag include having factory-sealed seams with straps made from reinforced material that are riveted (not sewn) and run along the underside of the bag to create a sling to prevent the handles being ripped when the bag is lifted. The zipper should be on top and have two zipper tabs to allow them to be locked together with a zip tie.

- The middle layer is heat-sealable material that has been specially designed for decedent containment. It requires a thermal sealer to seal the edges to create a pouch that will encapsulate the remains after they are placed in the first bag. This material comes with a factory-sealed edge that, when opened, one side can hang down the side of the gurney to protect it from the contaminated bed during transfer of the body into this bag. Any imprinted indicators on where to seal and cut this material should not be followed as these are for the primary purpose of the material and not for biocontainment needs.
  - The innermost layer and first bag to be used (to be placed on top of the other two bags) is a 6-mil thickness (152 micrometers) mortuary bag made from vinyl or other chlorine-free fluid-impermeable material with sealed seams and a zipper on top.
- Scissors to cut the raw edges of the second bag after it has been heat-sealed.
- A camera or other device to take a photo of the patient prior to being contained.
- EPA-approved disinfectant wipes.
- Hand sanitizer.
- Zip tie for locking the zipper tabs on the third bag.

The required equipment in the cold zone includes:

- A hospital gurney or mortuary stretcher.
- An adhesive-backed pouch to attach to the decontaminated body bag to contain any necessary documentation.
- Single-use (disposable) gloves with extended cuffs and a long-sleeved disposable gown.
- Spill kit with PPE and spill cleanup supplies.
- Infectious substance labels that are applied to the decontaminated body bag, including the following:
  - Black and white "infectious substance" label

- United Nations (UN) 2814 Category A infectious substance label
- "Do not open" label
- Label with the name and phone number of the hospital administrator

The CDC 21-step process is available at https://www.cdc.gov/vhf /ebola/clinicians/evd/handling-human-remains.html. Although other facilities may use slightly different processes, the process shown in this publication has been adapted to include additional considerations that have been used successfully in the Nebraska Biocontainment Unit (NBU; see table 20.1). The process involves taking the gurney with the preopened bags into the hot zone and positioning it alongside the bed and transferring the decedent into each bag while in the hot zone. Consideration should be given to cleaning and disinfecting the floor and taking measures to protect the gurney from coming into contact with any contaminated surfaces in the room prior to wheeling it in to lessen the potential for contamination.

The CDC guidelines can be adapted to meet the needs and physical layout of individual facilities. For example, the NBU process follows the CDC principles, but they developed a method that did not require taking the gurney with all three bags into the hot zone. The NBU facility utilizes an additional zone referred to as the warm zone, in which the remains are transferred after being contained in the second bag by using a slide board to create a bridge from the foot of the bed to the head of the gurney that has the third bag ready to receive the remains. This allows staff to slide the disinfected double-bagged remains directly into the heavy-duty mortuary bag. This same technique is then repeated at the transition between the warm and cold zones into a second heavy-duty mortuary bag. At each transfer, staff in appropriate PPE for their assigned zones take custody of the remains. The teams for this process in the NBU consist of up to 4 staff in the hot zone, 2 in the warm zone, and 2 in the clean (cold) zone.

Transportation of Infected Human Remains

The US Department of Transportation (DOT) regulates the transportation of infectious substances including HHCD-infected human remains (see chapter 19 on waste handling), which are categorized into two main groups: Category A and Category B infectious substance. A Category A infectious substance is defined as:

> A material known or reasonably expected to contain a pathogen, such as Ebola, that is in a form capable of causing permanent disability or life threatening or fatal disease in otherwise healthy humans or animals when exposed to it. (49 CFR, Parts 171–180)

Category B infectious substances are those that do not meet the criteria to be included in Category A and therefore do not require the same stringent measures as hazardous material. To determine the appropriate category for human remains, the DOT provides this guidance: "An infectious substance classification is based on the patient or animal's known medical history or symptoms, endemic local conditions, or professional judgment concerning the individual circumstances of the source human or animals." Using this definition it would appear that transporting Ebola-infected human remains would be subject to the requirements for transporting Category A infectious substances. However, if the remains are being transported for cremation, interment, or medical research, they are exempted from Hazardous Materials Regulations (HMR) 49 CFR, Parts 171–180. However, infectious substance labels must still be applied to the external mortuary bags. Once sealed within the mortuary bags, the remains can be transported in the same manner as any other decedent with some caveats. The transport route should be predetermined and arranged in collaboration with all relevant authorities, according to state regulations. Consideration should be given to limiting the transit time from the point of containment to the final destination, as well as how to maintain chain of custody during transit. If the transport route involves interstate travel, it must be coordinated with the CDC Emergency Operations Center (EOC). Finally, in the unlikely event a spill were to occur, the transportation team should have PPE readily available and be familiar with (or receive just-in-time training on) how to clean up a spill, and how to contain and dispose of the waste it will generate.

Support for Family and Friends

Family members and friends of patients who are in isolation are unlikely to have any physical contact with them during their illness. Visitation will be restricted to available resources, and at best communication will have been provided via two-way video connections. Although seeing a loved one on a screen is better than not seeing them at all, it does not replace the need to have direct physical or verbal contact when death is imminent. Visitation rules after the patient dies are unlikely to change, and being isolated from loved ones at times such as this can lead to a profound feeling of loss and helplessness. Supporting the family and making all attempts to comfort and provide what is required to help them cope during this period is a key element of preparedness that should be included in planning.

Each individual family will be unique in their needs, so it will be important to individualize support and assess their beliefs, which traditions they want to uphold and what needs are priorities for them. Many people have religious practices that are important at the time of death, so consideration should be given to facilitating these requests, when feasible. Using the video system to administer blessings is one way that can accommodate this need and will not place someone at risk with room entry. It may also be helpful to allow the family to write letters or provide other items such as photos that can be included when securing the decedent within the mortuary bags. This will give the family an opportunity to express their personal feelings and give them a sense of connection to their loved one.

Supporting Staff

In addition to the family, staff may also experience a sense of loss and perhaps failure at not being able to save their patient. At one US facility that experienced the death of an Ebola patient during the 2014 West Africa Ebola outbreak, a study that interviewed staff on their experience asked about the emotional impact of providing care to a patient with an HCCD. Fully half of these staff members reported that the death of their patient was the most difficult experience they encountered. To prepare staff to cope, it is beneficial to have a behavioral health specialist on the team who can provide counseling and a safe place for them to express their feelings, but also to provide resiliency training in advance of an event to prepare them to use preidentified resiliency strategies. It may also be helpful for them to acknowledge the decedent by memorializing them in some way. This can be done through having a meeting or service to honor the person and give staff the opportunity to express condolences. It is important to acknowledge that staff will find this an emotional event, and opportunities need to be provided to allow the healing process to begin.

Summary

The postmortem care of a patient must be performed with attention to detail and a high level of infection control. Leadership and staff should be knowledgeable about the regulations that govern the health and safety of the worker, as well as how the decedent should be contained and transported. Methods for containing the decedent can range from placing a mask over their airway to containing them in several layers of differing standards of mortuary bags following a detailed procedure. Transportation of an HCCD-infected decedent needs to follow DOT regulations. As with any death of a patient, it will be an emotional time for family, friends, and staff, so in addition to strict infection prevention and control measures, it is important not to lose sight of the need for emotional and spiritual support needs of those involved.

Table 20.1. Process for Handling of Human Remains

1. Prepare the thermal sealer by plugging it into an electrical outlet and placing it in a safe location to avoid inadvertent burns to staff. Ensure it is plugged in where it will allow the sealer to reach the entire circumference of the second bag.

2. Use the camera or other device to take a photograph of the decedent's face for identification purposes. Make sure to follow your facility's compliance regulations when digitally transfer-

ring the image to not violate the Healthcare Insurance Portability Accountability Act (HIPAA).

3. Position the gurney with the three preopened body bags next to the hospital bed. The overhanging top of the heat-sealable material should be positioned toward the bed to protect the gurney. It is also useful to remove the head and footboard from the bed as this will allow easier access to the body.

4. Do not remove any inserted medical devices such as an IV line or endotracheal tube from the body. Simply disconnect any equipment and move them away from the work area. Do not remove dressings. Do not wash or clean the body. Do wrap the bed linens around the body as this will help absorb any liquids as well as immobilize the extremities.

5. Gently roll the body from one side to the other to clean the bed with EPA-registered disinfectant wipes to remove any body fluids and lower the bio burden on the mattress. Allow the mattress to dry, then remove the first bag from the gurney. Gently roll the body wrapped in the linen to one side while sliding the first bag under the body, and positioning it so that when the body is rolled back it will be positioned in the center of the bag.

6. Once the body is positioned on the first bag, zip it up, being careful not to let anyone's gloves get caught in the zipper mechanism. Minimize the amount of air that will be trapped in the bag, as this will prevent a risk of aerosolizing pathogens when pressure is put on the bag during transfer.

7. Disinfect gloved hands using alcohol-based hand rub (ABHR) or EPA-registered disinfectant wipes after each step. If any areas of PPE have visible contamination, disinfect with an EPA-registered disinfectant wipe. Consider wearing a disposable apron over the PPE as this can be removed and replaced easily in the hot zone.

8. Disinfect the outside of the first bag with an EPA-registered hospital disinfectant applied according to the manufacturer's recommendations. If there is any body fluid from the patient on the bag, be sure to clean it first, then disinfect. Ensure adequate wetness, friction, and dry time are provided when disinfecting.

9. Transfer the first bag with the body in it to the gurney, placing it on top of the second bag material. Consider adding a slider board to the list of required equipment as this will assist with the transfer and reduce the risk of tearing the first bag when lifting it with the weight of the body inside.

10. Disinfect gloved hands using ABHR or EPA-registered disinfectant wipes. If wearing a disposable apron, remove it and don a clean one.

11. Fold the overhanging side of the second bag material over the first bag, and heat-seal approximately 2 inches around the entire perimeter. Although one edge is factory sealed, it should be resealed to mitigate complications from a potential factory defect in the sealing process. For additional safety, consider adding small clamps to the equipment list as they are useful for holding the material edges together during the sealing process, and will prevent having to place hands close to the thermal sealer. After sealing around the entire circumference, heat-seal the bag a second time approximately 1 inch below the initial seal and then heat-seal diagonally across the corners. Use scissors to trim the excess material by cutting down the center of the outermost seal. This will result in a perfectly sealed edge. Turn off and unplug the thermal sealer and place it in a safe location to cool. The thermal sealer must be decontaminated before being removed from the hot zone or reused.

12. Disinfect the outside of the second bag with an EPA-registered hospital disinfectant applied according to the manufacturer's recommendations. Be careful when wiping the edges, as they can be sharp.

13. Disinfect gloved hands using ABHR or EPA-registered disinfectant wipes.

14. Work the third bag around the second bag, and zip up the third bag, again being careful to not get any gloves caught in the zipper mechanism. When the zipper tabs meet, use a zip tie to lock them together.

15. Disinfect gloved hands using ABHR or EPA-registered disinfectant wipes. If wearing a disposable apron, remove it and don a clean one.

16. Wipe down the gurney with EPA-registered disinfectant, then wheel the gurney to the decontamination area for a more thorough cleaning and disinfection.

17. Decontaminate the surface of the body bag with an EPA-registered hospital disinfectant applied according to the manufacturer's recommendations. Begin by applying the hospital disinfectant to the top of the bag and any exposed areas of the gurney. Engage the side rail, then roll the bag to one side to decontaminate half of the bottom of the bag and the newly exposed portion of the gurney. Repeat with the other side of the bag and gurney. When performing decontamination, remove any visible soil on surfaces of the bag or gurney with the EPA-registered disinfectant wipes. After the visible soil has been removed, reapply the hospital disinfectant, and allow sufficient contact time as specified by the manufacturer of the disinfectant.

18. Disinfect the surfaces of the gurney from the handles to the wheels with an EPA-registered hospital disinfectant applied according to the manufacturer's recommendations.

19. Disinfect gloved hands using ABHR or EPA-registered disinfectant wipes.

20. Push the gurney gently so that only the gurney and the decontaminated body bag enter the cold zone. The workers in the

hot zone should not enter the cold zone. The cold zone team will receive the body and transport the body for disposition.

21. The hot zone team should proceed to the PPE doffing area and follow facility procedures for doffing PPE.

CHAPTER 21

Public Health Partnership

CAITLIN S. PEDATI

Isolation and quarantine orders can be important tools for protecting the public's health and controlling the spread of communicable diseases. As discussed in more detail in chapter 3, in the United States these functions are supported by legislation at the federal, state, and frequently local levels. It is important for personnel in the medical and public health fields to be aware of these laws and the means by which governmental public health officials can use them to support disease control and prevention of the spread of communicable diseases.

At the federal level, presidential executive orders are used to determine which diseases or conditions may justify the use of federal quarantine or isolation measures. The Centers for Disease Control and Prevention (CDC) has the authority to detain and subsequently assess detained persons, who may be suspected of having a quarantinable condition when they arrive at a US port of entry or travel between states. The CDC also plays a lead role in restricting or managing the movement of persons between states through activities such as placing individuals on the "Do Not Board" list or coordinating transport to another state for treatment of a particular condition. Additionally, the CDC's Division of Global Migration and Quarantine routinely provides monitoring and evaluation services for persons, remains, animals, or cargo products that could represent a risk to the public's health, and they can be called on to evaluate concerns identified and reported by airplane pilots or ship captains.

States have a similar role and the responsibility to contain and control the spread of communicable diseases within their borders. The specific diseases covered by quarantine and isolation orders can vary from state to state, as can the individual or agency responsible for issuing such orders and the repercussions for violating them. Each state maintains a list of reportable conditions that may vary from one jurisdiction to another, but reportable conditions are primarily used as epidemiologic tools for disease surveillance and don't necessarily equate to quarantinable conditions. However, when a clinician or laboratory reports a condition in accordance with state law, this could trigger the issuance of a quarantine or isolation order. Such orders might also be issued to address a known exposure to a communicable disease or a request for an evaluation of a concerning event, where multiple people who may have been exposed to a pathogen in a shared setting develop signs and symptoms of a communicable disease. Each state has legislation that identifies responsible parties with the authority to issue quarantine and isolation orders. Usually, this action can be performed by the governor, the state health officer, or medical director of the state board of health. Additionally, depending on the structure of the public health system in a given state, the director or board of health of a local health department may have similar authority to issue these orders within their jurisdiction. Most states indicate that these orders should be executed by the least restrictive means possible, and in many cases, the public health agency issuing the order assumes the responsibility of providing care and necessities such as lodging and food to persons under a quarantine or isolation order. An order might simply restrict a person from attending certain group activities, performing specific job duties, or being present in public settings; it could limit a person to their own home, or it may require coordination to admit a person to a health care facility or alternate housing option. Coordination with law enforcement agencies is sometimes required to execute these orders, and violations are considered a misdemeanor in most states.

Once an isolation or quarantine order is issued, there must also be a protocol in place for patient monitoring, as well as for the requirements that must be achieved in order to release a person from the order. Health departments can employ a variety of mechanisms to track individuals under an order and assess them for the development of symptoms, including in-person visits, phone calls, electronic survey applications, or video conferencing, depending on the disease and available resources. If an order is issued to quarantine or isolate a person who was exposed in a work setting, the occupational health division of a facility might also assist with such monitoring. Public health personnel should ensure that persons under quarantine or isolation orders have a good understanding of the specific movement restrictions that apply to them as well as when and how to seek care, if needed. This typically requires coordination among state and local public health partners as well as designated emergency services personnel and health care facilities and providers.

It is not unusual for an event that necessitates quarantine or isolation to involve governmental public health agencies at several levels. Effective and efficient communication and coordination among these different levels, between states/jurisdictions, and with key partners including laboratories, emergency services personnel, health care providers, and the general public is a critical component for executing quarantine and isolation orders effectively for the protection of the public's health.

CHAPTER 22

Clinical Research in the HLCC Setting

ELIZABETH R. SCHNAUBELT

COLLEEN S. KRAFT

Introduction

Providing safe and effective care to patients in a high-level containment care (HLCC) setting poses unique challenges to both clinicians and researchers. Diseases managed in the HLCC setting, particularly novel, rare, or emerging infectious diseases such as Ebola virus disease (EVD), often lack proven effective (licensed) therapeutic options. In addition, disease management may be challenged further by the lack of approved diagnostic tests. Furthermore, access to diagnostic equipment for clinical management may be limited by the risk of device contamination or inaccessibility of the device in an HLCC setting. Finally, effective screening and proven postexposure management strategies are limited in the absence of available opportunities to study novel and emerging infectious diseases in a rigorous scientific manner. Despite these challenges, the HLCC setting offers opportunities for clinical research to advance scientific knowledge amid a paucity of high-quality clinical data for certain special pathogens and emerging infectious diseases. Appropriately designed protocols are imperative to answer questions related to safety and efficacy of potential therapeutic interventions, diagnostics platforms, and prevention strategies, including vaccines.

Human Subjects' Protection and Good Clinical Practices in HLCC Clinical Research

It is important to distinguish between that which constitutes clinical care and those activities that constitute research in a patient care environment. Much of the care administered in an HLCC setting with the sole intention of enhancing the well-being of a patient is considered treatment within the context of medical practice. However, systematic data collection with the intent to develop or contribute to generalizable knowledge is research. The Office for Human Research Protections (OHRP) provides guidance to establish whether an activity is human subjects research, so clinicians can be mindful of their obligations to uphold the Belmont Report[1] ethical principles and follow guidelines for the protection of human subjects and comply with the US Department of Health and Human Services (HHS) Code of Federal Regulations (CFR) Title 45 Part 46 (45 CFR 46) Protection of Human Subjects.

Notably, the HHS Federal Policy for the Protection of Human Subjects, also known as the Common Rule, underwent revisions in 2017, and investigators conducting HHS-regulated research must comply with the new requirements as of January 21, 2019. The revised Common Rule contains significant updates including, among other changes, (1) new requirements regarding the information that must be given to prospective research subjects as part of the informed consent process; (2) allowing the use of broad consent (i.e., seeking prospective consent to unspecified research) from a subject for storage, maintenance, and secondary research use of identifiable private information and biospecimens; (3) establishing a requirement for US-based institutions engaged in cooperative research to use a single institutional review board (IRB) for the portion of the research that takes place within the United States, with certain exceptions.

Additional regulations related to clinical research and use of products regulated by the Food and Drug Administration (FDA) include 21

---

1 *The Belmont Report: Ethical Principles and Guidelines for the Protection of Human Subjects of Research, Report of the National Commission for the Protection of Human Subjects of Biomedical and Behavioral Research*, published in 1978 by the National Commission for the Protection of Human Subjects of Biomedical and Behavioral Research, is a widely accepted summary of the ethical principles of research in humans.

CFR 50 (Protection of Human Subjects), 21 CFR 56 (Institutional Review Boards), and 21 CFR 312 (Investigational New Drugs). These regulations allow for specific exemptions when conducting emergency research and may apply to clinical research in HLCC settings. Investigators conducting clinical research should adhere to the standards of good clinical practice as outlined in the International Council for Harmonization Integrated Addendum E6(R2) to E6(R1). It is ultimately the responsibility of the investigator to guarantee the safety and welfare of participants in clinical research and to ensure that study subjects are adequately protected while maintaining their rights, autonomy, and personal dignity.

Treatment Research: Investigational Therapeutics and Devices

In the absence of licensed therapies, clinicians caring for patients in an HLCC setting may seek use of investigational products that are in a preclinical or early clinical phase, and which have not yet been vetted through the lengthy drug development process and the scientific rigor of clinical trials. When considering use of an investigational drug or biological product, investigators must deliberate on and weigh the risk of potential harm against the potential benefit of an intervention to the subject. Ideally, an option with a favorable risk-benefit ratio can be determined prior to seeking use of an investigational therapeutic. Such an assessment may be particularly challenging when clinicians are faced with managing a life-threatening disease for which data regarding interventions are limited to preclinical trials and may not be publicly available.

Subpart I of 21 CFR 312 provides for expanded access to investigational drugs for treatment of immediately life-threatening conditions for which there is no comparable or satisfactory alternative therapy to diagnose, monitor, or treat the patient's disease or condition. Section 310 of this regulation delineates specifications for emergency use in individual patients, provided the physician determines that the probable risk to the person from the investigational new drug (IND) is not greater than the probable risk from the disease or condition and the FDA determines that the patient cannot obtain the drug under another IND or existing protocol. Treatment is generally limited to a single course of therapy for a specified duration unless the FDA expressly authorizes multiple courses or chronic therapy. The licensed physician or sponsor must explain how the expanded access use will meet the requirements of §§312.305 and 312.310 and must agree to submit an expanded access submission to the FDA within 15 working days of FDA's authorization of the use.

During the 2014–16 West Africa Ebola outbreak, 15 facilities in the United States and Europe provided care to 27 patients with EVD, 23 of whom received at least one investigational therapy. However, there were very limited data available to clinicians and researchers to guide the selection, administration, and monitoring of existing therapeutic options. In addition, lack of a coordinated research network led to institutions independently seeking the best available treatment options for their individual patients. The use of investigational therapeutics with heterogeneous clinical data collection and lack of standardized protocols across institutions limited the ability to make conclusions as to whether the therapeutic provided clinical benefit. In addition, use of multiple investigational therapeutics simultaneously precluded definitive conclusions related to efficacy or potential harm from any individual drug. Despite these limitations, data reported from these clinical observations can generate knowledge and can inform the design of future randomized clinical trials.

Investigational Devices

While providing HLCC care, lack of approved diagnostic tests may severely limit a clinician's ability to manage their patients appropriately. Use of a medical device that has not yet been approved or cleared by the FDA is considered investigational and generally should only be used in human subjects if it is approved for clinical testing under an investigational device exemption (IDE). Investigational devices, including in vitro diagnostic tests, may be considered for use in clinical care under the provisions of a treatment IDE if the device is intended to treat or diagnose a serious or immediately life-threatening disease or condition for which there is no comparable or satisfactory alternative device, the device is under investigation in a controlled clinical trial for the same use under an approved IDE, and the sponsor of the investigation is actively pursuing marketing approval/clearance of the investigational device with due diligence.

Additional Clinical Research Opportunities in a HLCC Unit

In addition to treatment research, HLCC offers critical opportunities in other areas of clinical research to enhance knowledge and understanding of novel and emerging infectious diseases. Such research may include diagnostics, screening and prevention research, disease natural history, and epidemiological studies.

Reliable diagnostic assays are critically important to identify individuals infected with a particular pathogen accurately and may be necessary to monitor their response to treatment. Often in the setting of an emerging infectious disease outbreak, diagnostic tests may be limited only to those available in research settings or reference laboratories, thus reducing a clinician's ability to make timely management decisions for their patients. During the care of the first patients with EVD in the United States, the Serious Communicable Diseases Unit at Emory University and the Nebraska Biocontainment Unit at the University of Nebraska Medical Center/Nebraska Medicine evaluated a diagnostic assay not yet approved for clinical use. This study demonstrated comparable performance of a research-use-only FilmArray® Biothreat-E panel when compared to the more complex molecular assays available at the time through the Centers for Disease Control and Prevention (CDC), suggesting a more accessible and easier-to-use assay with a rapid turnaround time. During the course of this study, the FDA subsequently issued an emergency use authorization (EUA) to allow use of this assay in the clinical setting.

Laboratory analysis of biospecimens during the course of a patient's illness may support findings from animal models and inform future preclinical research. Comprehensive laboratory investigations, such as kinetic analysis of biomarkers, can lead to basic science discovery and improved understanding of the pathogenesis of rare and emerging infectious diseases. A main challenge of these studies is the ability to perform these types of investigations with samples classified as Category A or select agents. These cannot be performed at the clinical institutions, and the shipping and storage of these is regulated by the Division of Select Agents and Toxins at the CDC. The sponsors of the investigational drug or devices may need to collaborate with a BSL-4–capable research laboratory to overcome some of the regulatory challenges.

Screening and prevention research should be prioritized in the midst of a public health emergency to identify potentially infected individuals accurately and to implement protective measures rapidly. Safe and effective pre- and postexposure prophylaxis options, such as vaccines, drugs, and biological products, are needed for individuals potentially exposed to Ebola virus or other special pathogens. Vaccine trials conducted during the West Africa Ebola outbreak provided vitally important data on vaccine safety and immunogenicity and informed the design and execution of future vaccine studies necessary to assess efficacy, including during later Ebola outbreaks in 2018 and 2019 in the Democratic Republic of the Congo.

Special Pathogens Research Network

The West Africa Ebola outbreak highlighted key gaps of research infrastructure necessary to implement scientifically sound, ethical clinical trials rapidly in the midst of a public health emergency. In response, the National Ebola Training and Education Center (NETEC), funded by the Assistant Secretary for Preparedness and Response (ASPR) and the CDC, established the Special Pathogen Research Network (SPRN) in collaboration with federal and academic partners to develop infrastructure for cohesive, coordinated clinical research efforts related to Ebola and other special pathogens. Key deliverables of the SPRN include creation of a master protocol for research, operationalization of a central IRB, development of universal case report forms, and web-based clinical data capture to facilitate collation and interpretation of data to inform clinical management, potentially in real time during an outbreak. The SPRN has established a medical countermeasures working group to develop guidance on therapeutics and prophylaxis measures, which will facilitate prompt and efficient awareness of potential investigational interventions. The SPRN is also developing a network biorepository focused on special pathogens with policies and procedures for processing and storage of specimens. A biorepository offers valuable opportunities for future research, particularly when the number of patients affected by rare and emerging infectious diseases enrolled in clinical research may be limited.

Practical Considerations

Even in state-of-the-art, well-resourced facilities, conducting clinical research in an HLCC unit poses significant challenges. There are practical considerations that investigators should anticipate in preparing for clinical research in such a setting. Ensuring that valid informed consent is obtained from a study participant, a critical component of human subjects protection, may be especially challenging when patients are suffering from a life-threatening illness for which there are no apparent alternative treatments. Patients who are critically ill may have decreased lucidity and awareness, rendering them unable to fully comprehend the proposed therapeutic benefit and potential associated risks of an investigational therapy. In such circumstances, or in other situations when a patient is unable to consent for themselves, locating a legally authorized representative in a timely fashion within a potentially narrow therapeutic window may be difficult. Finally, there may also be challenges communicating effectively with patients during the informed consent process simply due to personal protective equipment (masks, PAPRs) causing sound muffling.

Documenting informed consent and maintaining other source documents in an HLCC setting may pose added challenges. Inability to fully decontaminate items from a patient care area may render use of paper documents impractical or prohibitive. Investigators may utilize alternate means, such as electronic documentation or photographs of documents that may be securely transmitted from a contaminated area, as long as the IRB is made aware of and approves of this plan.

A sponsor of an investigational therapeutic may require specific monitoring procedures, such as electrocardiograms, or serial laboratory tests that are not readily available or accessible. Investigators should develop policies and procedures to safely conduct necessary monitoring as required by the sponsor, but investigators and the sponsor should also consider which interventions are absolutely required versus optional to minimize risks to patients and staff alike.

Finally, health care workers providing HLCC to a patient may not be trained in clinical research. Conversely, research staff may not have prior experience with high-level personal protective equipment (PPE) to safely operate in an HLCC environment. Investigators may seek staff who have experience or familiarity with both clinical research and HLCC operations. Alternatively, research staff may receive just-in-time PPE training for safe and effective interaction in the HLCC unit, or provide training to HLCC health care workers on good clinical practices and protection of human subjects to conduct clinical research.

Reporting and Dissemination of Findings

Investigators conducting clinical research must comply with reporting requirements to the IRB, the FDA, and the sponsor. In addition, timely data sharing and dissemination of findings are critical to advance scientific knowledge and inform future investigations rapidly. In some cases, knowledge gained in real time could have an invaluable impact on the care of other patients during an outbreak. One must also consider the crucial aspect of respecting the privacy of the individual in the reporting, given that the number of cases evaluated may be few. This can be accomplished by obtaining consent from the individual, who may agree to the dissemination of their information, or by publishing in aggregate reports that include results from other patients or studies. In September 2015 the World Health Organization (WHO) convened a consultative meeting of international stakeholders to promote the sharing of data and results during public health emergencies. The WHO subsequently published a statement encouraging researchers in both public and private sectors to share data and quality-controlled preliminary results to advance public health, prevent illness, and save lives. Several prominent journals concurred in a consensus statement declaring that journals should encourage public sharing of relevant data and that authors should not be penalized for sharing data in the interest of resolving an urgent situation prior to manuscript submission.

Conclusion

In summary, clinical research is an important element in the management of patients cared for in the HLCC setting, especially when there are no licensed interventions. Knowledge gained, if managed effectively, has the potential to improve the care of subsequent patients, even as the outbreak unfolds. Research in this setting provides additional challenges, above and beyond the usual challenges of conducting clinical research, related to obtaining patient consent, managing records, collecting laboratory specimens, and maintaining patient confidentiality. However, by being prepared in advance to conduct research efficiently and in the spirit of collaboration, researchers can provide significant benefit to patients immediately and in the long term.

REFERENCES AND ADDITIONAL RESOURCES

Chapter 1

Centers for Disease Control and Prevention. History of quarantine. https://www
.cdc.gov/quarantine/historyquarantine.html. Last updated January 10, 2012.
Accessed May 31, 2019.

Rosenberger LH, Riccio LM, Campbell KT, et al. Quarantine, isolation, and cohorting: From cholera to *Klebsiella*. *Surg Infect.* 2012;13(2):69–73.

Tognotti E. Lessons from the history of quarantine, from plague to influenza A.
Emerg Infect Dis. 2013;19(2):254–259.

Chapter 2

Department of Health and Human Services, Office of the Assistant Secretary for
Preparedness and Response. *Regional Treatment Network for Ebola and
Other Special Pathogens.* https://www.phe.gov/Preparedness/planning/hpp
/reports/Documents/RETN-Ebola-Report-508.pdf. Published November
2017. Accessed May 31, 2019.

National Association of County and City Health Officials. CDC announces new
preparedness brief and Ebola treatment hospitals. https://www.naccho.org
/preparedness-brief/cdc-announces-ebola-treatment-hospitals-and-new
-interim-hospital-guidance. Published December 2, 2014. Accessed May 31,
2019.

National Ebola Training and Education Center. *Annual Report FY2018.* https://
netec.org/wp-content/uploads/2019/01/NETEC-Annual-Report-FY2018.pdf.
Published 2019. Accessed May 31, 2019.

US Department of Health and Human Services. *Hospital Preparedness Program
(HPP) Measure Manual: Implementation Guidance for Ebola Preparedness
Measures.* https://www.phe.gov/Preparedness/planning/sharper/Documents
/hpp-mmi-guide-ebola-508.pdf. Published May 2017. Accessed May 31, 2019.

Chapter 3

Katz R, Vaught A, Formentos A, Capizola J. Raising the yellow flag: State variation in quarantine laws. *J Pub Health Manag Pract.* 2018;24(4):380–384.

Misrahi JJ. The CDC's communicable disease regulations: Striking the balance between public health and individual rights. *Emory L J.* 2018;67(3):463–488.

Chapter 4

Cieslak TJ, Herstein JJ, Kortepeter MG. Communicable diseases and emerging pathogens: The past, present, and future of high-level containment care. In Hewlett A, Murthy ARK, eds. *Preparing for Bioemergencies: A Guide for Healthcare Facilities.* New York: Springer, 2018:1–20.

Chapter 5

Centers for Disease Control and Prevention. Quarantine and isolation. https://www.cdc.gov/quarantine/index.html. Last updated September 29, 2017. Accessed May 31, 2019.

University of Nebraska Medical Center. Global center for health security: About page. https://www.unmc.edu/healthsecurity/about/index.html. Accessed May 31, 2019.

Chapter 6

Centers for Disease Control and Prevention. Identify, isolate, inform: Emergency department evaluation for patients under investigation (PUI) for Ebola virus disease (EVD). https://www.cdc.gov/vhf/ebola/clinicians/emergency-services/emergency-departments.html. Last updated March 22, 2016. Accessed May 31, 2019.

Koenig KL. Identify, isolate, inform: A 3-pronged approach to management of public health emergencies. *Disaster Med Public Health Prep.* 2014;9(1):86–87.

Schwedhelm S, Swanhorst J, Watson S, Rudd J. ED Ebola triage algorithm: A tool and process for compliance. *J Emerg Nurs.* 2015;41(2):165–169.

Schwedhelm SS, Wadman MC. Process development for the care of the person under investigation for Ebola virus disease: A collaboration of biocontainment unit and emergency medicine personnel. *Curr Treat Option Infect Dis.* 2016; doi: 10.1007/s40506-016-0099-z.

Wadman MC, Schwedhelm SS, Watson S, et al. Emergency department processes for the evaluation and management of persons under investigation for Ebola virus disease. *Ann Emerg Med.* 2015;66(3):306–314.

Chapter 7

American Institute of Architects. Guidelines for Design and Construction of Hospital and Health Care Facilities. https://www.fgiguidelines.org/wp-content /uploads/2016/07/2006guidelines.pdf. Published 2006. Accessed May 31, 2019.

Centers for Disease Control and Prevention. Guidelines for preventing the transmission of *Mycobacterium tuberculosis* in health-care settings. *MMWR.* 2005;54(RR-17):1–141.

Siegel JD, Rhinehart E, Jackson M, Chiarello L, and the Healthcare Infection Control Practices Advisory Committee. *2007 Guidelines for Isolation Precautions: Preventing Transmission of Infectious Agents in Healthcare Settings.* https:// www.cdc.gov/infectioncontrol/pdf/guidelines/isolation-guidelines-H.pdf. Last updated May 2019. Accessed May 31, 2019.

Chapter 8

Bannister B, Puro V, Fusco FM, et al. Framework for the design and operation of high-level isolation units: Consensus of the European Network of Infectious Diseases. *Lancet Infect Dis.* 2009;9(1):45–56.

Beam E, Gibbs SG, Hewlett AL, et al. Clinical challenges in isolation care. *Am J Nurs.* 2015;115(4):44–49.

Centers for Disease Control and Prevention. Guidance on personal protective equipment (PPE) to be used by healthcare workers during management of patients with confirmed Ebola or persons under investigation (PUIs) for Ebola who are clinically unstable or have bleeding, vomiting, or diarrhea in U.S. hospitals, including procedures for donning and doffing PPE. https://www .cdc.gov/vhf/ebola/healthcare-us/ppe/guidance.html. Last updated August 30, 2018. Accessed May 31, 2019.

Smith PW, Anderson AO, Christopher GW, et al. Designing a biocontainment unit to care for patients with serious communicable diseases: A consensus statement. *Biosecur Bioterror.* 2006;4(4):351–365.

Smith PW, Boulter KC, Hewlett AL, et al. Planning and response to Ebola virus disease: An integrated approach. *Am J Infect Control.* 2015;43(5):441–446.

Chapter 9

Cates DS, Gomes PG, Krasilovsky, AM. Behavioral health support for patients, families, and healthcare workers. In Hewlett A, Murthy ARK, eds. *Bio-emergency Planning: A Guide for Healthcare Facilities*. Cham, Switzerland: Springer, 2018:195–214.

Chopra V, Flanders SA, Saint S, et al. Michigan Appropriateness Guide for Intravenous Catheters (MAGIC) Panel. *Ann Intern Med*. 2015;163(6 Suppl):S1–40.

Chapter 10

Centers for Disease Control and Prevention. Interim guidance for U.S. hospital preparedness for patients under investigation (PUIs) or with confirmed Ebola virus disease (EVD): A framework for a tiered approach. https://www.cdc.gov/vhf/ebola/healthcare-us/preparing/hospitals.html. Last updated August 30, 2018. Accessed May 31, 2019.

Hewlett AL, Varkey JB, Smith PW, Ribner BS. Ebola virus disease: Preparedness and infection control lessons learned from two biocontainment units. *Curr Opin Infect Dis*. 2015;28(4):343–348.

Kortepeter MG, Bausch DG, Bray M. Basic clinical and laboratory features of filoviral hemorrhagic fever. *J Infect Dis*. 2011;204(Suppl 3):S810–816.

Kortepeter MG, Smith PW, Hewlett A, Cieslak TJ. Caring for Ebola patients: A challenge in any care facility. *Ann Int Med*. 2015;162(1):68–69.

Uyeki TM, Mehta AK, Davey RT, et al. Clinical management of Ebola virus disease in the United States and Europe. *N Engl J Med*. 2016;374(7):636–646.

Chapter 11

Arabi YM, Balkhy HH, Hayden FG, et al. Special report: Middle East respiratory syndrome. *N Engl J Med*. 2017;376(6):584–594.

Alraddadi BM, Al-Salmi HS, Jacobs-Slifka K, et al. Risk factors for Middle East respiratory syndrome: Coronavirus infection among healthcare personnel. *Emerg Infect Dis*. 2016;22(11):1915–1920.

Centers for Disease Control and Prevention. Infection Control for Prehospital Emergency Medical Services (EMS). 2005. Available at: https://www.cdc.gov/sars/guidance/i-infection/prehospital.html.

Centers for Disease Control and Prevention. Guidance on Air Medical Transport for Middle East Respiratory Syndrome (MERS) Patients. 2017. Available at: https://www.cdc.gov/coronavirus/mers/hcp/air-transport.html.

Centers for Disease Control and Prevention. Guidance on Air Medical Transport for SARS Patients. 2005. Available at: https://www.cdc.gov/sars/travel/airtransport.html.

Cowling BJ, Jin L, Lau EHY, et al. Comparative epidemiology of human infections with avian influenza A H7N9 and H5N1 viruses in China: A population-based study of laboratory-confirmed cases. *Lancet.* 2013;382(9887):129–137.

Gao H-N, Lu H-Z, Cao B, et al. Clinical findings in 111 cases of influenza A (H7N9) virus infection. *N Engl J Med.* 2013;368(19):2277–2285.

Hayden F, Croisier A. Transmission of avian influenza viruses to and between humans. *J Infect Dis.* 2005;192(8):1311–1314.

Peiris JS, Yuen KY, Osterhaus SD, Stohr K. The severe acute respiratory syndrome. *N Engl J Med.* 2003;349(25):2431–2441.

Tan CC. SARS in Singapore: Key lessons from an epidemic. *Ann Acad Med Singapore.* 2006;35(5):345–349.

Varia M, Wilson S, Sarwal S, et al. Investigation of a nosocomial outbreak of severe acute respiratory syndrome (SARS) in Toronto, Canada. *CMAJ.* 2003;169(4):285–292.

Yu ITS, Li Y, Wong TW, et al. Evidence of airborne transmission of the severe acute respiratory syndrome virus. *N Engl J Med.* 2004;350(17):1731–1739.

Chapter 12

Barquet N, Domingo P. Smallpox: The triumph over the most terrible of the ministers of death. *Ann Int Med.* 1997;127(8 Pt 1):635–642.

Breman JG, Henderson DA. Diagnosis and management of smallpox. *N Engl J Med.* 2002;346(17):1300–1308.

Casey CG, Iskander JK, Roper MH, et al. Adverse events associated with smallpox vaccination in the United States, January–October 2003. *JAMA.* 2005;294(21):2734–2743.

Fleischauer AT, Kile JC, Davidson M, et al. Evaluation of human-to-human transmission of monkeypox from infected patients to health care workers. *Clin Infect Dis.* 2005;40(5):689–694.

Grosenbach DW, Honeychurch K, Rose EA, et al. Oral tecovirimat for the treatment of smallpox. *N Eng J Med.* 2018;379(1):44–53.

Henderson DA, Inglesby TV, Bartlett JG, et al. Smallpox as a biological weapon. *JAMA.* 1999;281(22):2127–2137.

Jezek Z, Grab B, Szczeniowski MV, et al. Human monkeypox: Secondary attack rates. *Bull WHO.* 1988;66(4):465–470.

McCollum AM, Damon IK. Human monkeypox. *Clin Infect Dis.*
2014;58(2):260–267.

Nalca A, Rimoin AW, Bavari S, Whitehouse CA. Reemergence of monkeypox: Prevalence, diagnostics, and countermeasures. *Clin Infect Dis.*
2005;41(12):1765–1771.

Reynolds MG, Yorita KL, Kuehnert MJ, et al. Clinical manifestations of
human monkeypox influenced by route of infection. *J Infect Dis.*
2006;194(6):773–780.

Sepkowitz KA. How contagious is vaccinia? *N Eng J Med.* 2003;348(5):439–446.

Wehrle PF, Posch J, Richter KH, Henderson DA. An airborne outbreak of smallpox in a German hospital and its significance with respect to other recent
outbreaks in Europe. *Bull WHO.* 1970;43(5):669–679.

Chapter 13

Arunkumar G, Chandni R, Mourya DT, et al. Outbreak investigation of Nipah
virus disease in Kerala, India. *J Infect Dis.* 2018; doi: 10.1093/infdis/jiy612.

Baussano I, Nunn P, Williams B, et al. Tuberculosis among health care workers.
Emerg Infect Dis. 2011;17(3):488.

Epstein J, Field H, Luby S, et al. Nipah virus: Impact, origins, and causes of emergence. *Curr Infect Dis Rep.* 2006;8(1):59–65.

Kool JL. Risk of person-to-person transmission of pneumonic plague. *Clin Infect
Dis.* 2005;40(8):1166–1172.

Chapter 14

Centers for Disease Control and Prevention. Guidelines for preventing the transmission of *Mycobacterium tuberculosis* in health-care settings. *MMWR.*
2005;54(RR-17):1–141.

Fiebelkorn AP, Redd SB, Kuhar DT. Measles in healthcare facilities in the United States during the post-elimination era, 2001–2014. *Clin Infect Dis.*
2015;61(4):615–618.

Humphreys H. Control and prevention of healthcare-associated tuberculosis: The
role of respiratory isolation and personal respiratory protection. *J Hosp
Infect.* 2007;66(1):1–5.

Shenoi SV, Escombe AR, Friedland G. Transmission of drug-susceptible and
drug-resistant tuberculosis and the critical importance of airborne infection

control in the era of HIV infection and highly active antiretroviral therapy
rollouts. *Clin Infect Dis.* 2010;50(Suppl 3):S231–7.

Siegel JD, Rhinehart E, Jackson M, Chiarello L, and the Healthcare Infection
Control Practices Advisory Committee. Guideline for isolation precautions:
Preventing transmission of infectious agents in healthcare settings (2007).
https://www.cdc.gov/infectioncontrol/guidelines/isolation/index.html. Last
updated May 24, 2019. Accessed May 31, 2019.

Chapter 15

Gangarosa EJ, Barker WH. Cholera: Implications for the United States. *JAMA.*
1974;227(2):170–171.

Roberts J. Quarantine or isolation in diphtheria? *J Am Pub Health Assoc.*
1911;1(5):353–358.

Chapter 16

Cieslak T, Evans L, Kortepeter M, et al. Perspectives on the management of children
in a biocontainment unit: Report of the NETEC Pediatric Workgroup.
Health Security. 2019;17(1):11–17.

Chapter 17

Centers for Disease Control and Prevention. Guidance for collection, transport and
submission of specimens for Ebola virus testing. https://www.cdc.gov/vhf
/ebola/laboratory-personnel/specimens.html. Last updated May 15, 2018.
Accessed May 31, 2019.

Centers for Disease Control and Prevention. Guidance for U.S. laboratories for
managing and testing routine clinical specimens when there is a concern
about Ebola virus disease. https://www.cdc.gov/vhf/ebola/laboratory
-personnel/safe-specimen-management.html. Last updated June 1, 2018.
Accessed May 31, 2019.

Centers for Disease Control and Prevention. Interim biosafety guidance for all
individuals handling clinical specimens or isolates containing 2009-H1N1 influenza A virus (Novel H1N1), including vaccine strains. https://www.cdc.gov
/h1n1flu/guidelines_labworkers.htm. Published August 15, 2009. Accessed
May 31, 2019.

Centers for Disease Control and Prevention. Interim laboratory biosafety guidelines for handling and processing specimens associated with Middle Eastern respiratory syndrome coronavirus (MERS-CoV), version 2. https://www.cdc.gov/coronavirus/mers/guidelines-lab-biosafety.html. Last updated September 14, 2017. Accessed May 31, 2019.

Iwen PC, Alter R, Herrera VL, et al. Laboratory processing of specimens. In Hewlett A, Murthy K, Rekha A, eds. *Bioemergency Planning*. Cham, Switzerland: Springer, 2018:67–82.

Chapter 18

Biselli R. Aeromedical evacuation of patients with hemorrhagic fevers: The experience of Italian Air Force aeromedical isolation team. *J Hum Virol Retrovirol*. 2015; doi: 10.15406/jhvrv.2015.02.00058.

Centers for Disease Control and Prevention. Guidance for developing a plan for interfacility transport of persons under investigation or confirmed patients with Ebola virus disease in the United States. https://www.cdc.gov/vhf/ebola/clinicians/emergency-services/interfacility-transport.html. Last updated January 28, 2016. Accessed May 31, 2019.

Centers for Disease Control and Prevention. Sample: Standard operating procedure (SOP) for decontamination of an ambulance that has transported a patient under investigation or patient with confirmed Ebola. https://www.cdc.gov/vhf/ebola/clinicians/emergency-services/ambulance-decontamination.html. Last updated January 28, 2016. Accessed May 31, 2019.

Christopher GW, Eitzen EM, Jr. Air evacuation under high-level biosafety containment: The aeromedical isolation team. *Emerg Infect Dis*. 1999;5(2):241–46.

Coignard-Biehler H, Isakov A, Stephenson J. Pre-hospital transportation in Western countries for Ebola patients, comparison of guidelines. *Intensive Care Med*. 2015;41(8):1472–1476.

Ewington I, Nicol E, Adam M, et al. Transferring patients with Ebola by land and air: The British military experience. *J Royal Army Med Corps*. 2016;162(3):217–221.

Isakov A, Jamison A, Miles W, Ribner B. Safe management of patients with serious communicable diseases: Recent experience with Ebola virus. *Ann Intern Med*. 2014;161(11):829–830.

Isakov A, Miles W, Gibbs S, et al. Transport and management of patients with confirmed or suspected Ebola virus disease. *Ann Emerg Med.* 2015;66(3):297–305.

Klaus J, Gnirs P, Holterhoff S, et al. Disinfection of aircraft: Appropriate disinfectants and standard operating procedures for highly infectious diseases. *Bundesgesundheitsblatt-Gesundheitsforschung-Gesundheitsschutz.* 2016;59(12):1544–1548.

Lowe JJ, Jelden KC, Schenarts PJ, et al. Considerations for safe EMS transport of patients infected with Ebola virus. *Prehosp Emerg Care.* 2015;19(2):179–183.

Chapter 19

Bibby K, Fischer RJ, Casson LW, et al. Disinfection of Ebola virus in sterilized municipal wastewater. *PLoS Negl Trop Dis.* 2017; doi: 10.1371/journal.pntd.0005299.

Lowe JJ, Gibbs SG, Schwedhelm SS, et al. Nebraska Biocontainment Unit perspective on disposal of Ebola medical waste. *Am J Infect Control.* 2014;42(12):1256–1257.

Chapter 20

Centers for Disease Control and Prevention. Guidance for safe handling of human remains of Ebola patients in U.S. hospitals and mortuaries. https://www.cdc.gov/vhf/ebola/healthcare-us/hospitals/handling-human-remains.html. Last updated February 11, 2015. Accessed May 31, 2019.

Prescott JB, Bushmaker T, Fischer RJ, et al. Postmortem stability of Ebola virus. *Emerg Infect Dis.* 2015;21(5):856–859.

Smith M, Smith PW, Kratochvil C, Schwedhelm M. The psychosocial challenges of caring for patients with Ebola virus disease. *Health Security.* 2017;15(1):104–109.

Chapter 21

Centers for Disease Control and Prevention. Quarantine and isolation. https://www.cdc.gov/quarantine/index.html. Last updated September 29, 2017. Accessed May 31, 2019.

National Conference of State Legislatures. State quarantine and isolation statutes. http://www.ncsl.org/research/health/state-quarantine-and-isolation-statutes .aspx. Published October 29, 2014. Accessed May 31, 2019.

Chapter 22

Federal Register. *Federal Policy for the Protection of Human Subjects.* https://www .federalregister.gov/documents/2017/01/19/2017-01058/federal-policy-for-the -protection-of-human-subjects. Published January 19, 2017. Accessed May 31, 2019.

Mendoza EJ, Qui X, Kobinger GP. Progression of Ebola therapeutics during the 2014–2015 outbreak. *Trends Mol Med.* 2016;22(2):164–172.

Uyeki TM, Mehta AK, Davey RT Jr, et al. Clinical management of Ebola virus disease in the United States and Europe. *N Engl J Med.* 2016;374(7):636–646.